普通高等教育"十三五"规划教材　配套实验与学习指导系列
全国高等医药院校规划教材

医学组织学
图谱与实习指导

ATLAS OF MEDICAL HISTOLOGY AND PRACTICAL GUIDE

王大亮　周德山　郭晓霞　徐　健　主编
Wang Daliang　Zhou Deshan　Guo Xiaoxia　Xu Jian

清华大学出版社
北京

内 容 简 介

《医学组织学图谱与实习指导》是针对医学组织学课程专门编写的教材。本教材主要介绍人体基本组织及各器官在光学显微镜下的细微结构、电子显微镜下的超微结构以及相应的形态学特征。全书共分为19章，每个章节分别设定学生观察切片及示教切片不同内容。同学们可以根据章节的学习目的和要求，掌握重点的组织学结构及形态特征知识，同时结合思考题和临床内容联系知识点的练习对所学知识进行巩固及拓展。

本教材为中英双语教材，有利于培养同学们的英语应用能力，也有助于国际学生的组织学课程的学习。图片中增加了电镜、特殊染色以及免疫荧光染色的图片类型，有利于同学们更清楚地观察组织结构的细微特点。本教材可供高等院校医学专业及相关学科的学生和科研人员使用和参考。

Introduction

Atlas of Medical Histology and Practucal Guide is a textbook specially compiled for medical histology courses. This textbook is focused on the microstructure of the human tissues and organs under the light microscopy, the ultrastructure under the electron microscopy and the corresponding morphological characteristics. The textbook is divided into 19 chapters. Each chapter contains observation sections and teaching sections. Matching the objectives and requirements of each chapter, students can master the key knowledge of histological structure and morphological characteristics, and at the same time, consolidate and expand the knowledge by incorporating the questions and clinical correlations sections.

The textbook is bilingual in Chinese and English, which will facilitate English application and international students to learn histology course. The included electron microscope, special staining and immunofluorescence staining pictures will help students to observe more differential characteristics of histological structure. This textbook can also be used as a reference book for medical students and researchers in colleges and universities.

图书在版编目（CIP）数据

医学组织学图谱与实习指导 / 王大亮等主编 . — 北京：清华大学出版社，2019（2025.3 重印）
（普通高等教育"十三五"规划教材　全国高等医药院校规划教材配套实验与学习指导系列）
ISBN 978-7-302-52380-2

Ⅰ．①医… Ⅱ．①王… Ⅲ．①人体组织学 – 医学院校 – 教学参考资料 Ⅳ．① R32

中国版本图书馆 CIP 数据核字（2019）第 037586 号

责任编辑：罗　健　周婷婷
封面设计：常雪影
责任校对：刘玉霞
责任印制：宋　林

出版发行：清华大学出版社
　　　　　网　　址：https://www.tup.com.cn, https://www.wqxuetang.com
　　　　　地　　址：北京清华大学学研大厦A座　　　　　邮　　编：100084
　　　　　社总机：010-83470000　　　　　　　　　　　邮　　购：010-62786544
　　　　　投稿与读者服务：010-62776969, c-service@tup.tsinghua.edu.cn
　　　　　质量反馈：010-62772015, zhiliang@tup.tsinghua.edu.cn
印 装 者：三河市龙大印装有限公司
经　　销：全国新华书店
开　　本：185mm×260mm　　　印　　张：12　　　字　　数：302千字
版　　次：2019年9月第1版　　　　　　　　　　　印　　次：2025年3月第5次印刷
定　　价：69.80元

产品编号：065654-01

编 委 会
Editorial Board

前 言

组织学是以形态学为主的医学基础课，内容上主要介绍人体四种基本组织及各器官在光学显微镜（简称"光镜"）下的细微结构、电子显微镜（简称"电镜"）下的超微结构以及相应的形态学特征。在学习过程中辅以大量的组织学图片，有利于学生更好地掌握组织学知识。

为响应教育部双语教学的号召，顺应医学教育国际化发展的趋势，本教材采用中英文两种语言，有利于学生们在掌握组织学知识的同时，加深对专业英语词汇的掌握。为了使本教材中的医学组织学专业术语更加规范，特邀请美国凯撒研究所的病理学专家朱立青博士对本书的英文内容进行审校，并邀请北京大学医学部组织学与胚胎学教研室主任张宏权教授对本书的中文内容进行了审核。

除了上述中英双语的主要特点之外，本教材还有以下几个特点：①书中图片经过了精心筛选，既包含彩色的光镜图片和电镜图片，也包含免疫荧光、特殊染色等类型的图片，图文并茂。②在每个章节的前面，有关于重点知识的简要介绍，在章节的后面有思考题，有利于学生把握章节的要点。③每个章节后面有适当的知识拓展阅读材料，为教师的教学和学生的学习提供了丰富的辅助资料。④本书的结尾有英-中文组织学名词对照索引，有利于满足学生在学习时查阅的需求。⑤本书配有思考题答案，便于学生加深对知识的理解。

本教材根据全国普通高等教育"十三五"国家级规划教材教学大纲编写，由清华大学、首都医科大学、北京大学医学部三家医学院校的教师共同完成。

本教材全面而系统地精选了包括光镜、电镜以及免疫荧光、特殊染色等共 294 幅图片，并进行了详细的注解。

在编写本教材的过程中，清华大学出版社、清华大学教务部门给予了大力支持，在此深表谢意！

由于水平有限，书中难免存在不尽如人意之处，因此，非常期待老师和同学们的批评和建议。

王大亮

2019 年 3 月于清华园

PREFACE

Medical histology is a morphology-based medical branch, which studies basic tissue components and various organ systems in human body, including micro-structure under light microscopy, and ultrastructure under electron microscopy, as well as the corresponding morphological characters. Studying images/micrographs is essential in understanding the morphology.

Given the need of internationalization of medical education, our national ministry of education has called upon bilingual teaching. Written in both Chinese and English, this text and atlas is aimed at helping students master knowledge of histology and build medical vocabulary in English at the same time. We thus invited, Dr. Zhu Lee-Ching, a senior pathologist and researcher at Kaiser Permanente -Washington and Kaiser Research Institute in U.S. to proofread the text in English. We also invited Professor Zhang Hongquan, director of department of Histology and Embryology in Peking University Health Science Center, reviewed the Chinese contents of this text book.

This *Atlas of Medical Histology and Practical Guide* is carefully designed. We selected combined images of light micrographs, electron micrographs as well as images of immunofluorescence, immunohistochemical and special staining to reflect the frontier development of modern histology. The sections of "Objectives" and "Questions" are helpful for students to grasp important studying points and directions. The section of "Correlations with Clinic and Scientific Research" provides abundant ancillary materials for further teaching and studying. The "Vocabulary index" at the end of this text book, provides an easy access to the study material.

This text book is prepared according to the national 13th five-year plan for teaching outline of *Histology and Embryology*, with the collaboration of Tsinghua University School of Medicine, Peking University Health Science Center and Capital Medical University.

A total of 294 images, including images of light microscope, electron microscope, immunofluorescence and special stains, are selected carefully in this text book, and are marked in detail.

We gratefully acknowledge the help of Tsinghua University Press and Tsinghua University education department, for their great support in the publication.

We would greatly appreciate any comments or suggestions regarding the book *Atlas of Medical Histology and Practical Guide*.

Wang Daliang, March, 2019 on Tsinghua campus

目 录

CONTENTS

第1章 细 胞

Chapter 1 Cell

【实习内容】Contents of Observation

示教图片 Teaching Pictures

1. 细胞核	1. Nucleus
2. 粗面内质网与核糖体	2. Rough endoplasmic reticulum & ribosome
3. 滑面内质网	3. Smooth endoplasmic reticulum
4. 高尔基复合体	4. Golgi complex
5. 溶酶体	5. Lysosome
6. 线粒体	6. Mitochondrion
7. 过氧化物酶体	7. Peroxisome
8. 微丝（肌动蛋白丝）	8. Microfilament（actin filament）
9. 微管	9. Microtubule
10. 中心体	10. Centrosome
11. 脂滴	11. Lipid droplet
12. 糖原颗粒	12. Glycogen particle
13. 细胞周期	13. Cell cycle

【目的要求】

1. 掌握细胞核、细胞膜的结构及组成。
2. 掌握细胞质内细胞器的组成、电镜结构特点。
3. 熟悉细胞骨架的组成及结构特点。
4. 了解染色体的核型、染色质／染色体的变化特点。
5. 了解细胞周期、细胞分裂过程及各阶段的细胞形态特点。

【Objective】

1. To master the structure and composition of cell nucleus and membrane.

2. To master the composition of the cytoplasmic organelles and their features under electron microscopy (EM).

3. To be familiar with the composition and structure of the cytoskeleton.

4. To understand the characteristics of chromosome karyotype, changes of chromatin / chromosome.

5. To understand the cell cycle, cell division and their morphological characteristics at different stages.

【示教图片】
【Teaching Pictures】

❶ 图片 1：细胞核

图 1-1a（电镜，EM）显示细胞核中淡染均质区域为常染色质（1），深染区域为异染色质（2），核中央为核仁（3）。图 1-1b 显示核外周为核膜部分，核膜为双层膜结构，核内膜（1）与核外膜（2）由核周腔（3）相分隔。核膜上有许多核孔（4），介导细胞核与细胞质之

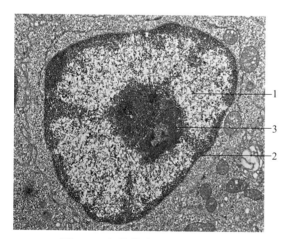

图 1-1a 细胞核（EM，12 000×）
Fig.1-1a Nucleus (EM, 12 000×)

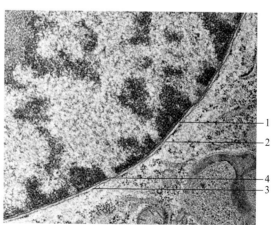

图 1-1b 核膜与核孔（EM，30 000×）
Fig.1-1b Nuclear membrane and pores
(EM, 30 000×)

间的物质交换。

1. Picture 1: Nucleus

Figure 1-1a (Electronic Microscope, EM) shows the pale-stained homogenous region as euchromatin (1) and dark-stained region as heterochromatin (2) in the nucleus. The nucleolus is located in the nucleus center (3). Figure 1-1b shows peripheral nucleus membrane as bilayer membrane structure. The inner membrane (1) and the outer membrane (2) were separated by the perinuclear cisterna (3). There are many nuclear pores (4) that allow the exchange of material between nucleus and cytoplasm.

② 图片 2：粗面内质网与核糖体

图 1-2 显示细胞核（1）周围，粗面内质网（2）为一膜性网状结构，其膜表面附有核糖体（3）。细胞质内也有游离的核糖体（4）存在。

2. Picture 2: Rough endoplasmic reticulum (RER) & ribosome

Figure 1-2 shows that around the nucleus (1), RER (2) is a membrane network structure that has ribosomes (3) attached to the cytoplasmic surface. Ribosomes also exist in cytoplasm (4).

③ 图片 3：滑面内质网

图 1-3 显示滑面内质网为细胞质内膜性网状结构，其表面没有核糖体附着。

3. Picture 3: Smooth endoplasmic reticulum (SER)

Figure 1-3 shows the SER is a membrane network structure in the cytoplasm which contains no ribosomes attached to its cytoplasmic surface.

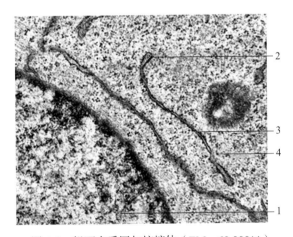

图 1-2　粗面内质网与核糖体（EM，60 000×）

Fig.1-2　RER and Ribosomes (EM, 60 000×)

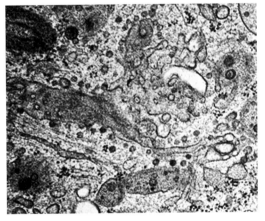

图 1-3　滑面内质网（EM，40 000×）

Fig.1-3　SER (EM, 40 000×)

④ 图片 4：高尔基复合体

图 1-4 显示高尔基复合体为膜性网状结构，由扁平囊重叠排列。高尔基复合体存在凸面（顺面）（1）和凹面（反面）（2），凸面接受粗面内质网新合成的囊泡（3），凹面将加工修饰的蛋白质浓缩小泡（4）释放出来。

4. Picture 4: Golgi complex

Figure 1-4 shows that the Golgi complex is a membrane network structure, which is arranged in an overlapped flat saccule. Golgi complex has cis-face (1) and trans-face (2). The former receives vesicles newly synthesized by RER (3), and the latter releases the modified protein condensing vacuoles (4).

❺ 图片5：溶酶体

初级溶酶体外有单层膜包被，色泽均匀，染色深。图1-5显示次级溶酶体（1）形态可有不同，内含物（2）色泽不均匀。残余体也称三级溶酶体。

5. Picture 5: Lysosome

A primary lysosome is enclosed by one membrane and has homogeneous, electron-dense granularity in its lumen. Figure 1-5 shows a secondary lysosome (1), which has partly digested material (2) in its lumen. Residual body is also named tertiary lysosome.

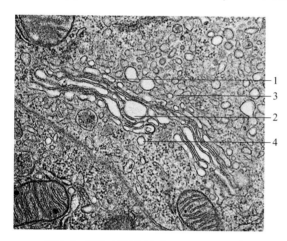
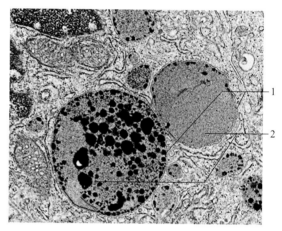

图1-4　高尔基复合体（EM，50 000×）

Fig. 1-4　Golgi complex (EM, 50 000×)

图1-5　次级溶酶体（EM，20 000×）

Fig. 1-5　Secondary lysosome (EM, 20 000×)

❻ 图片6：线粒体

线粒体截面呈圆形、椭圆形或哑铃状等，图1-6显示由外膜（1）、内膜（2）、膜间隙（3）和基质（4）组成。线粒体内膜向内突出形成线粒体嵴（5），嵴的横切面可呈囊状、管状或板层状。细胞质内见粗面内质网（6）和核糖体（7）。

6. Picture 6: Mitochondria

Cross sections of mitochondria are round, ovoid or dumbbell shapes. Figure 1-6 shows that the mitochondrion consists of an outer membrane (1), inter membrane (2), intermembrane space (3) and matrix compartment (4). The inner membrane projects into the mitochondrial matrix and forms the mitochondrion cristae (5), which show as cystic, tubular or lamellar shapes at transection sections. RER (6) and ribosomes (7) are in the cytoplasm.

❼ 图片7：过氧化物酶体

图1-7显示过氧化物酶体（1），含有精细的颗粒基质（2）和晶体核心（3）。

7. Picture 7: Peroxisomes

Figure 1-7 shows peroxisomes (1), which contain a finely granular matrix (2) and a crystalline core (3).

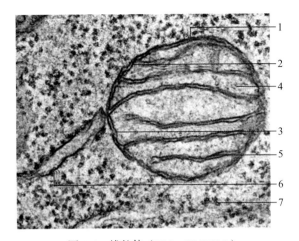

图 1-6 线粒体（EM，50 000×）

Fig. 1-6 Mitochondria (EM, 50 000×)

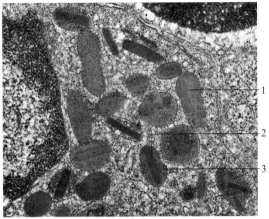

图 1-7 过氧化物酶体（EM，60 000×）

Fig. 1-7 Peroxisomes (EM, 60 000×)

⑧ 图片 8：微丝（肌动蛋白丝）

图 1-8 显示小肠微绒毛的纵切面。微绒毛（1）为细胞膜和细胞质共同伸出的指状突起，含有肌动蛋白丝（2）构成的致密结构轴心。

8. Picture 8: Microfilament (Actin filaments)

Figure 1-8 shows the longitudinal sections of the microvilli of small intestine. Microvilli (1), protrusions of plasma membrane, contain dense axis composed of actin filaments (2).

⑨ 图片 9：微管

微管是细长中空的圆柱形直管。微管蛋白为球形二聚体，先装配成原纤维，再由 13 条原纤维平行排列成单微管（1）（图 1-9a），特殊结构可存在二联微管和三联微管。图 1-9b 显示在培养中的细胞用抗 α- 微管蛋白抗体和 DAPI（2-（4- 氨基苯基）-6- 吲哚甲酰胺二盐酸盐，细胞核染色液）进行荧光免疫染色后，微管（红色）在细胞质中的分布。细胞核显示为蓝色。

9. Picture 9: Microtubule

Microtubule shows as a slender hollow cylindrical tube. Tubulin is spherical dimer,

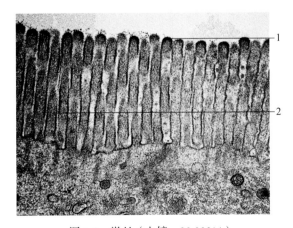

图 1-8 微丝（电镜，20 000×）

Fig. 1-8 Microfilament (EM, 20 000×)

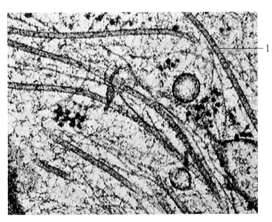

图 1-9a 微管（电镜，100 000×）

Fig. 1-9a Microtubule (EM, 100 000×)

assembled into fibrils, and then 13 fibrils arranged in parallel which form a single microtubule (1) (Figure 1-9a). Special structure can exist as double microtubules and triple microtubules. Figure 1-9b shows that immunofluorescent staining with anti-α-tubulin and DAPI (2- (4-Amidinophenyl) -6-indolecarbamidine dihydrochloride, nuclear staining solution) for cultured cells, the microtubules (red) extend throughout the cytoplasm. Nucleus is blue.

⑩ 图片10：中心体

图 1-10 显示细胞核周围一对相互垂直的中心粒（1）结构。中心粒为低柱状，由9组三联微管（2）组成。中心粒与其周围的细胞基质共同组成中心体。有丝分裂过程中，中心体通过微管蛋白的聚合，参与纺锤体等结构的形成。

10. Picture 10: Centrosome

Figure 1-10 shows a pair of centrioles (1), which are oriented perpendicular to each other around cell nucleus. Each comprise a ring of nine sets of fused microtubule triplets (2). The centrioles and pericentriolar matrix compose of centrosome. In mitosis, centrosome involves in the development of the mitotic spindle by polymerization of tubulin.

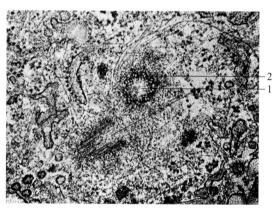

图 1-9b　微管（免疫荧光染色，400×）
Fig. 1-9b　Microtubule (IF, 400×)

图 1-10　中心体（电镜，100 000×）
Fig. 1-10　Centrosome (EM, 100 000 ×)

⑪ 图片11：脂滴

电镜下，脂滴为大小不等的泡状结构，没有界膜包绕，内容物一般为均质状，每个脂滴的电子密度不一，与脂滴的大小、内容物的性质以及固定染色的方法有关。图 1-11a 显示应用苏丹Ⅲ染色，细胞内的脂滴（1）呈橘黄色；图1-11b（电镜）显示肝细胞内呈球状的脂滴（1）。

11. Picture 11: Lipid droplet

In EM, lipid droplets are vesicular structures in varying sizes, with no membrane, and have homogeneous content. Its electron density varies, which is related to the size of the droplet, the content, as well as the method of fixation and staining. Figure 1-11a shows lipid droplets (1) in the cytoplasm as orange by Sudan Ⅲ staining; Figure 1-11b (EM) shows the spherical lipid droplets (1) in a hepatocyte.

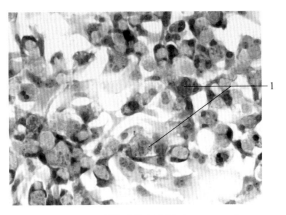

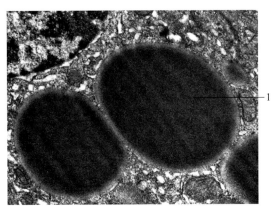

图 1-11a　脂滴（苏丹Ⅲ染色，200×）

Fig. 1-11a　Lipid droplet (Sudan Ⅲ staining)

图 1-11b　脂滴（电镜，10 000×）

Fig. 1-11b　Lipid droplet (EM, 10 000×)

⑫ 图片 12：糖原颗粒

糖原在通常切片中不易被观察，光镜下往往应用过碘酸 - 雪夫染色（图 1-12a，PAS 染色），显示为细胞内粉紫色结构（1）。电镜下，糖原颗粒无界膜包绕，电子密度比较高，形状不规则。图 1-12b 显示肝细胞内，糖原（1）形成较大颗粒成簇存在。

12. Picture 12: Glycogen granules

Glycogen is not usually seen in routine sections. In light microscopy (LM), the glycogen is shown as pink-purple (1) by periodic acid-Schiff staining (PAS staining, Figure 1-12a). In EM, glycogen appears as nonmembrane-bound, higher electron-dense granules with an irregular shape. In liver cells, they (1) often form larger, rosette-like aggregates (Figure 1-12b).

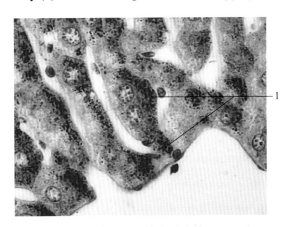

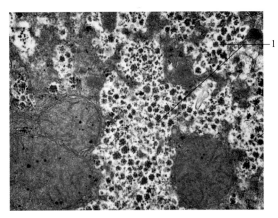

图 1-12a　糖原 PAS 染色（光镜，400×）

Fig. 1-12a　Glycogen PAS staining (LM, 400×)

图 1-12b　糖原颗粒（电镜，25 000×）

Fig. 1-12b　Glycogen granule (EM, 25 000×)

⑬ 图片 13：细胞周期

细胞周期指细胞从一次分裂完成开始到下一次分裂结束所经历的全过程，分为间期与分裂期两个阶段。间期分为静止期（G_0 期）、DNA 合成前期（G_1 期）、DNA 合成期（S 期）与DNA 合成后期（G_2 期）；分裂期又分为前期、中期、后期和末期四期。图 1-13（免疫荧光染色）显示细胞分裂的部分时期，α- 微管蛋白抗体和 DAPI 进行染色后，对比其他核蛋白染色

（绿色），微管定位于细胞质，并显示为红色，细胞核显示为蓝色。

13. Picture 13: Cell cycle

Cell cycle is the whole process from the conclusion of one cell division to the end of next cell division. Its two major phases are interphase and mitosis. The interphase comprises a quiescence (G_0 phase), DNA pre-synthesis (G_1 phase), DNA synthesis (S phase), and DNA post-synthesis (G_2 phase). Mitosis is divided into prophase, metaphase, anaphase and telophase. Figure 1-13 (Immunofluorescence, IF) shows a part of phases of cell cycle, in which microtubule is stained as red, and the nucleus as blue.

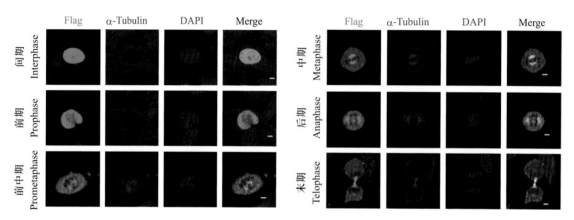

图 1-13　细胞周期（免疫荧光染色，630×）

Fig. 1-13　Cell cycle (IF, 630×)

【思考题】

1. 细胞质内常见的细胞器有哪些？其各自的主要功能是什么？
2. 什么是细胞骨架？其主要结构的基本组成及功能是什么？
3. 常染色质与异染色质的区别是什么？
4. 细胞周期包括哪些阶段？

【Questions】

1. Please list the common cell organelles, and describe their main functions respectively.

2. What is the cytoskeleton? Describe its basic compositions and function.

3. What is the difference between eurochromatin and heterochromatin?

4. What are the stages of a cell cycle?

【临床与科研联系英文阅读材料】
【English Reading Material for Correlations with Clinic and Scientific Research】

Mitochondrial encephalomyopathy, abbreviated to MELAS (Mitochondrial Encephalopahy,

Lactic Acidosis and Stroke-like episodes), is one of the family of mitochondrial cytopathies, which also include MERRF (Myoclonic Epilepsy with Ragged Red Fibers) and LHON (Leber's Hereditary Optic Neuropathy). It was first characterized under this name in 1984. A feature of these diseases is that they are caused by defects in the mitochondrial genome which is inherited purely from the female parent; however, it is important to know that some of the proteins essential to normal mitochondrial function are produced by the nuclear genome, and are subsequently transported to the mitochondria for use. As such, mutations in these proteins can result in mitochondrial disorders, but can be inherited from both male and female parents in the conventional fashion. The disease can manifest in both sexes. MELAS is a condition that affects many of the body's systems, particularly the brain and muscular system (encephalo-myopathy). MELAS is caused by mutations in the genes in mitochondrial DNA.

（李 英 王大亮）

第2章 上皮组织

Chapter 2 Epithelial Tissue

【实习内容】Contents of Observation

切片　Sections

观察切片	Observation Sections
1. 肠系膜铺片	1. Stretched preparation of mesentery
2. 回肠	2. Ileum
3. 肾	3. Kidney
4. 小肠	4. Small intestine
5. 气管	5. Trachea
6. 食管	6. Esophagus
7. 膀胱（空虚、充盈）	7. Urinary bladder（undistended, distended）

【目的要求】

1. 掌握上皮组织的一般结构特点和分类。
2. 掌握各种被覆上皮的结构特点和分布，在光镜下正确辨认各种被覆上皮。

【Objective】

1. To master structural characteristics and classification of the epithelial tissue.

2. To master structural features and distribution of different kinds of covering epithelia, and correctly identify them under the light microscopy.

【观察切片】
【Observation Sections】

① 切片 1：单层扁平上皮 – 铺片

材料与方法：动物肠系膜，硝酸银染色。

高倍镜观察：图 2-1 显示间皮细胞呈不规则的多边形，边缘呈黑色或棕色锯齿状。细胞质（1）呈深棕色；细胞核（2）呈圆形或椭圆形，居细胞中央，呈透明状。

1. Section 1: Simple squamous epithelium- stretched preparation

Materials and methods: Animal mesentery, silver nitrate staining.

HPM (High Power Magnification): Figure 2-1 shows that the mesothelial cells are polygonal in shape and the cell boundary is irregular, stained black or brown. The cytoplasm (1) is brown and the spherical or oval nuclei (2) are normally centrally positioned and transparent.

② 切片 2：单层扁平上皮 – 切片

材料与方法：动物回肠，HE 染色。

高倍镜观察：图 2-2，在粉红色的小肠壁外表面为单层扁平上皮（间皮）（1），可见细胞核呈扁椭圆形，着色深。细胞界限不清楚。

2. Section 2: Simple squamous epithelium-section

Materials and methods: Animal ileum, HE staining.

HPM: In Figure 2-2, the simple squamous epithelial cells/mesothelial cells (1) are found on the outside of the pink ileum. The nuclei are flatten and dark staining. The cell boundary is not clear.

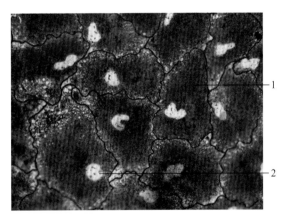

图 2-1　单层扁平上皮——铺片（400×）

Fig. 2-1　Simple squamous epithelium-
stretched preparation (400×)

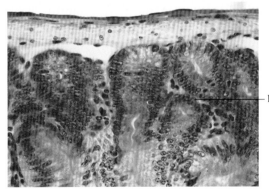

图 2-2　单层扁平上皮——切片（400×）

Fig. 2-2　Simple squamous epithelium-section (400×)

③ 切片 3：单层立方上皮

材料与方法：人肾，HE 染色。

高倍镜观察：图 2-3，管壁浅染，由一层近似立方形细胞（1）组成。核圆形，染成紫蓝色，位于细胞中央。

3. Section 3: Simple cuboidal epithelium

Materials and methods: Human kidney, HE staining.

HPM: The Figure 2-3 shows that the wall of the light stained tubule in the medulla consists of a single layer of cuboidal cells (1). The nucleus is spherical, central-located, and stained purple blue.

④ 切片 4：单层柱状上皮

材料与方法：动物小肠，HE 染色。

高倍镜观察：图 2-4 显示小肠绒毛表面被覆单层柱状上皮，可见柱状细胞（1）和杯状细胞（2）。柱状细胞呈高柱状，细胞核长椭圆形，位于细胞近基底部；细胞游离面为纹状缘（3）。杯状细胞散在于柱状细胞之间，细胞顶部膨大呈空泡状，底部狭窄，含深染的核。

4. Section 4: Simple columnar epithelium

Materials and methods: Animal small intestine, HE staining.

HPM: Figure 2-4 shows that the intestinal villus surface is covered by simple columnar epithelium, which consists of columnar cells (1) and goblet cells (2). The nucleus of the tall columnar cell is long ovoid and located toward the base of the cell. A thin, red-staining striated border (3) can be found on the free surface of the cell. Goblet cells lie between the columnar cells. The goblet cell has a broad apical portion and a narrow base. The dark-staining nucleus is ovoid or flat and located in the base of the cell.

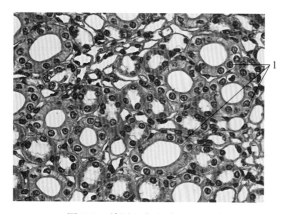

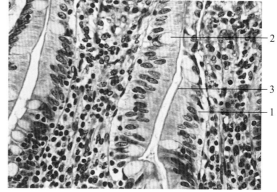

图 2-3　单层立方上皮（400×）
Fig. 2-3　Simple cuboidal epithelium (400×)

图 2-4　单层柱状上皮（400×）
Fig. 2-4　Simple columnar epithelium (400×)

⑤ 切片 5：假复层纤毛柱状上皮

材料与方法：人气管，HE 染色。

高倍镜观察：图 2-5，气管内表面被覆假复层纤毛柱状上皮，可见柱状细胞（1），细胞顶部较宽而基底部较窄，游离面可见染成浅红色的纤毛（2）；核椭圆形，位于细胞近游离面。锥形细胞（3）位于上皮基部，胞体较小，呈锥体形；核圆形，染色较深。杯状细胞（4）位于其他上皮细胞之间，与小肠柱状上皮内的杯状细胞相似。基膜（5）与上皮的基底面相贴，为均质状粉红色薄膜。

5. Section 5: Pseudostratified ciliated columnar epithelium

Materials and methods: Human trachea, HE staining.

HPM: In the Figure 2-5, the pseudostratified ciliated columnar epithelium is seen on the inner surface of tracheal wall. Note the apical portion of columnar cells (1) is slightly wider than the base.Light staining cilia (2) can be found on the free surface of the cell. The nucleus is ellipse and located near the apical part of the cell. Cone cells (3) are small pyramidal cells located at the base of the epithelium. The nucleus of cone cell is round, dark-staining. Goblet cells (4) lie among the other types of epithelial cells. The structure of goblet cell here is similar to that in small intestine simple columnar epithelium. Basement membrane (5), which is a pink-staining and homogenous thin layer, sticks underneath the epithelial cells.

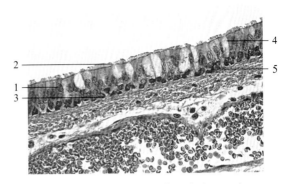

图 2-5　假复层纤毛柱状上皮（400×）

Fig. 2-5　Pseudostratified ciliated columnar epithelium (400×)

6 切片 6：复层扁平上皮

材料与方法：人食管，HE 染色。

低倍镜观察：图 2-6a 显示复层扁平上皮（1）由多层细胞密集排列形成。基底面（2）凹凸不平，可见结缔组织呈乳头状突入上皮（3）。

高倍镜观察：图 2-6b，基底层（1）为一层立方或低柱状细胞，细胞界限不清，胞质嗜碱性较强。中间层（2）为数层多边性细胞，细胞界限清楚，核圆形，位于中央。表层（3）有数层细胞，细胞呈扁平状；核扁，较小，染色深。

6. Section 6: Stratified squamous epithelium

Materials and methods: Human esophagus, HE staining.

LPM: In Figure 2-6a, the cells in stratified squamous epithelium (1) are arranged in more than one layer. The basal surface (2) of the epithelium is irregular, and the connective tissue papillae (3) bulge into the epithelium.

HPM: In Figure 2-6b, the basal layer (1) contains a layer of cuboidal or low columnar cells with

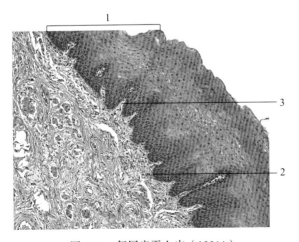

图 2-6a　复层扁平上皮（100×）

Fig. 2-6a　Stratified squamous epithelium (100×)

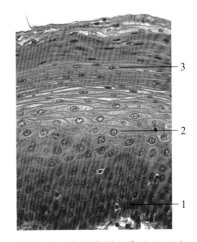

图 2-6b　复层扁平上皮（400×）

Fig. 2-6b　Stratified squamous epithelium (400×)

strong basophilic cytoplasm and ovoid nucleus. The cell boundaries are not clear. The intermediate layer (2) contains many layers of polygonal cells with distinct intercellular borders. The nucleus is spherical and central-located. The surface layer (3) contains several layers of flattened cells, with small flat dark-staining nucleus.

❼ 切片 7：变移上皮

材料与方法：动物膀胱，HE 染色。

低倍镜观察：图 2-7a 显示膀胱空虚状态，可见上皮（1）较厚，由多层细胞组成。图 2-7b 显示膀胱扩张状态，上皮（1）较薄，细胞层数少。两种状态的上皮表面均与基底面平行。

高倍镜观察：图 2-7c 显示膀胱空虚状态，表层细胞较大，又称盖细胞（1），胞质嗜酸性。中间层（2）为数层多边形细胞，核呈椭圆形。基底层（3）为一层立方形或低柱状细胞，核圆形，位于细胞中央。图 2-7d 显示膀胱扩张状态，盖细胞变扁呈梭形，核扁圆，其他各层细胞呈多边形，形状不一。

7. Section 7: Transitional epithelium

Materials and methods: Animal urinary bladder, HE staining.

LPM: Figure 2-7a shows undistended bladder. The epithelium (1) is thicker, with more layers of cells. The Figure 2-7b shows distended bladder. The epithelium (1) is thinner, with fewer layers of

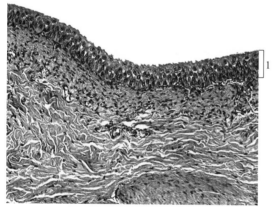

图 2-7a 变移上皮（空虚状态，100×）
Fig. 2-7a Transitional epithelium (Undistended, 100×)

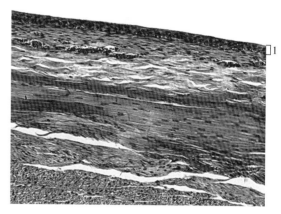

图 2-7b 变移上皮（扩张状态，100×）
Fig. 2-7b Transitional epithelium (Distended, 100×)

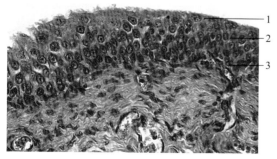

图 2-7c 变移上皮（空虚状态，400×）
Fig. 2-7c Transitional epithelium (Undistended, 400×)

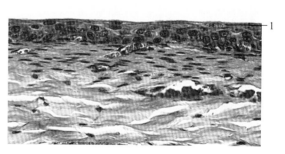

图 2-7d 变移上皮（扩张状态，400×）
Fig. 2-7d Transitional epithelium (Distended, 400×)

cells. The free surface of the epithelium parallels to the basement membrane.

HPM: Figure 2-7c shows undistended bladder. The superficial layer of the epithelium contains large cuboidal cells and multinucleated umbrella cells (1) with round nucleus and acidophilic cytoplasm. The intermediate layer (2) contains several layers of polygonal cells with oval nucleus. The basal layer (3) contains one layer of cuboidal or low columnar cells with central-located spherical nucleus. The Figure 2-7d shows distended bladder: The superficial (umbrella) cells become stretched and spindle in shape. The nucleus is flattened. The other cells are polygonal.

【作业】

绘图描述小肠单层柱状上皮高倍镜结构。

【Assignment】

Draw and describe morphological structures of small intestine simple columnar epithelium under high power microscopy.

【思考题】

1. 何谓上皮细胞的极性？其都有哪些特化结构？
2. 试述假复层纤毛柱状上皮的结构特点。
3. 如何区别复层扁平上皮和变移上皮？

【Questions】

1. What is the polarity of epithelial cells? What are the special structures included?
2. Try to describe the structural features of pseudostratified ciliated columnar epithelium.
3. How to distinguish stratified squamous epithelium from transitional epithelium?

【临床与科研联系英文阅读材料】
【English Reading Material for Correlations with Clinic and Scientific Research】

The stability and integrity of epithelial structure is an important guarantee for epithelial tissue to complete life activities. The epithelial-mesenchymal transition (EMT) is a highly networked cellular process which involves cell transition from the relatively immotile epithelial to the more motile mesenchymal phenotype, whereby cells lose their cell-cell adhesion and cell polarity and gain of migratory and invasive traits. EMT is essential for embryogenesis, fibrosis, tissue repair, wound healing, and tumor progression. Under pathological conditions, EMT occurs at the initial stage of cancer metastasis.

（郭晓霞　尚宏伟）

第3章 结缔组织

Chapter 3 Connective Tissue

【实习内容】Contents of Observation

 切片 Sections

观察切片	Observation Sections
1. 肠系膜铺片	1. Stretched preparation of mesentery
2. 疏松结缔组织（胃底）	2. Loose connective tissue（gastric fundus）
3. 不规则致密结缔组织（指皮）	3. Irregular dense connective tissue（finger skin）
4. 脂肪组织（指皮）	4. Adipose tissue（finger skin）
5. 网状组织（淋巴结）	5. Reticular tissue（lymph node）
示教切片	Teaching Sections
6. 成纤维细胞（肉芽组织）	6. Fibroblast（granulation tissue）
7. 规则致密结缔组织（肌腱）	7. Regular dense connective tissue（tendon）
8. 浆细胞	8. Plasma cell
9. 网状纤维（淋巴结）	9. Reticular fiber（lymph node）

【目的要求】

1. 掌握疏松结缔组织的形态和结构。
2. 了解致密结缔组织的形态特点。
3. 了解脂肪组织和网状组织结构和组成。

【Objective】

1. To master the morphology and structure of loose connective tissue.

2. To understand the morphological characteristics of dense connective tissue.

3. To understand the structure and composition of adipose tissue and reticular tissue.

【观察切片】
【Observation Sections】

❶ 切片 1：肠系膜铺片

材料与方法：大鼠肠系膜铺片。将台盼蓝注入大鼠的腹腔，次日处死大鼠，取其肠系膜，固定后，偶氮焰红和醛品红染色。

低倍镜观察：选择标本平整的部位观察，可见染成蓝色的细胞和红色及紫色的纤维。

高倍镜观察：图 3-1，观察巨噬细胞、肥大细胞、胶原纤维和弹性纤维的形态特点。肥大细胞（1）呈卵圆形，细胞质嗜碱性颗粒较密集，蓝色深染。巨噬细胞（2）吞噬了台盼蓝颗粒，颗粒大小不均，相对疏松。胶原纤维（3）被染成红色，纤维较粗大。弹性纤维（4）被染成紫色，呈细丝状，有分支。

1. Section 1: Stretched preparation of mesentery

Materials and methods: Rat stretched preparation of mesentery. 24 hours after trypan blue intraperitoneal injection, the rat was killed to collect the mesentery for aldehyde-fuchsin staining.

LPM: To observe blue cells, pink and purple fibers at the flat areas.

HPM: In the Figure 3-1, the morphological characters of macrophages, mast cells, collagenous fibers and elastic fibers were observed. The oval mast cells (1) have plenty of basophilic stippling in plasma. The macrophages (2) phagocytosed the granules of trypan blue, which were uneven in size, relatively loose. Collagen fibers (3) were stained pink and thick. Elastic fibers (4) are stained purple, with finely filamentous branches.

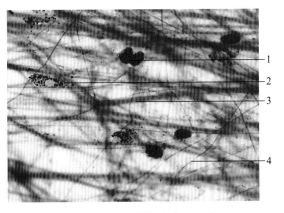

图 3-1　肠系膜铺片（400×）

Fig. 3-1　Stretched preparation of mesentery (400×)

❷ 切片 2：疏松结缔组织（胃底）

材料与方法：人胃底，HE 染色。

低倍镜观察：图 3-2a，黏膜下层中的疏松结缔组织，细胞（1）稀少，细胞间质发达，血管（2）较多，可看见胶原纤维（3）的各种断面。

高倍镜观察：图 3-2b 示不同走行方向的纤维断面。

2. Section 2: Loose connective tissue (gastric fundus)

Materials and methods: Human gastric fundus, HE staining.

LPM: Figure 3-2a shows that the loose connective tissue is located in the submucosal layer. There are few cells (1) and ample stroma with plenty of blood vessels (2). Collagen fibers are irregular (3).

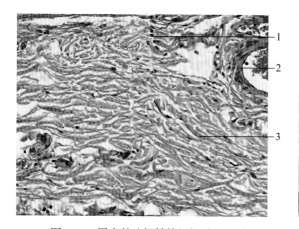

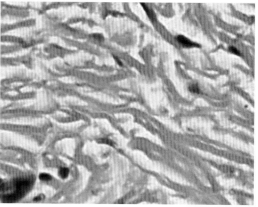

图 3-2a 胃底的疏松结缔组织（100×）

Fig. 3-2a Loose CT in the submucosa of stomach (100×)

图 3-2b 胃底的疏松结缔组织（400×）

Fig. 3-2b Loose CT in the submucosa of stomach (400×)

HPM: The Figure 3-2b shows the different shapes and directions of the fibers.

❸ 切片 3：不规则致密结缔组织（指皮）

材料与方法：人指皮，HE 染色。

低倍镜观察：图 3-3a 显示皮肤真皮部分。可见粗大、密集的胶原纤维（1）和少量的细胞（2）。

高倍镜观察：图 3-3b，纤维（1）不规则，可见有各种走行方向和断面。

3. Section 3: Irregular dense connective tissue（finger skin）

Materials and methods: Human finger skin, HE staining.

LPM: Figure 3-3a shows that the dermis of the skin of the abdominal wall consists of the massive thick dense collagen fibrils (1) and small amounts of cells (2).

HPM: Figure 3-3b shows that the irregular dense connective tissue fibers (1) present with the different directions and shapes of collagen fibrils.

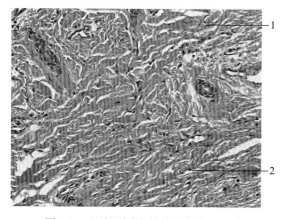

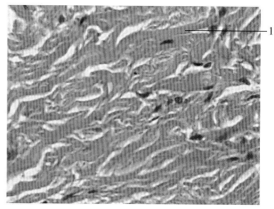

图 3-3a 不规则致密结缔组织（100×）

Fig. 3-3a Irregular dense connective tissue (100×)

图 3-3b 不规则致密结缔组织（400×）

Fig. 3-3b Irregular dense connective tissue (400×)

④ 切片 4：脂肪组织（指皮）

材料与方法：人指皮，HE 染色。

低倍镜观察：图 3-4a 显示皮肤皮下组织，可见脂肪组织中脂肪细胞（1）成群分布，被疏松结缔组织（2）分成许多脂肪小叶。

高倍镜观察：图 3-4b，脂肪细胞的形态。单泡脂肪细胞（1）密集成群，细胞体积较大，呈球形或者多边形。细胞中间为一个大脂滴（在制作切片过程中被溶解掉）呈空泡状，细胞质被挤到细胞周边。细胞核呈扁圆形，位于细胞一侧，形似戒指。

4. Section 4: Adipose tissue (finger skin)

Materials and methods: Human finger skin, HE staining.

LPM: Figure 3-4a shows the subcutaneous tissue of the finger skin. The adipocytes (1) are in lobulated distribution, surround by the loose connective tissue (2).

HPM: Figure 3-4b shows the morphological characteristics of adipocytes. Unilocular adipocytes (1) are densely arranged in connective tissue. These spherical and polyhedral adipocytes are large. The lipid droplet in the center of cells has been dissolved in organic solvent during the section preparation. The nucleus and cytoplasm of adipose cells are pushed under the membrane like a thin ring.

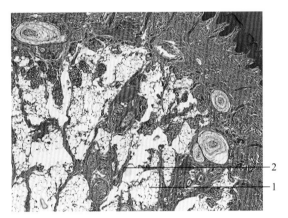 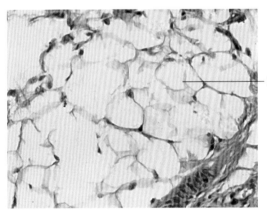

图 3-4a　脂肪组织（100×）
Fig. 3-4a　Adipose tissue (100×)

图 3-4b　脂肪组织（400×）
Fig. 3-4b　Adipose tissue (400×)

⑤ 切片 5：网状组织（淋巴结）

材料与方法：人淋巴结，HE 染色。

低倍镜观察：图 3-5a 显示人淋巴结。周围染色较深，为皮质（1），中间染色浅，为髓质（2）。髓质内的髓质淋巴窦（3），细胞成分较少。

高倍镜观察：图 3-5b，淋巴结髓质淋巴窦内的各细胞成分：网状细胞、淋巴细胞、巨噬细胞。网状细胞（1），细胞核卵圆形，染色浅，核仁明显。淋巴细胞（2）的细胞核呈圆形，染色深，胞质少。静止期的巨噬细胞（3）呈圆形或卵圆形，细胞质嗜酸性强。

5. Section 5: Reticular tissue (lymph node)

Materials and methods: Human lymph node, HE staining.

LPM: Figure 3-5a shows a human lymph node. The peripheral area of lymph node is deep stained, which is the cortex (1), the center of lymph node is lighter stained, which is the medulla (2). Pay attention to the lymphoid sinus of the medulla, where the cellularity is less condense.

HPM: Figure 3-5b shows variable cells in the medullary lymphoid sinus, including reticular cells, lymphocytes and macrophages. The reticular cells (1) are characteristically ovoid, lighter stained, with distinct nucleoli. Lymphocytes (2) have spherical and deep stained nuclei, with little cytoplasm. The macrophages (3) generally contain spherical or ovoid nuclei and the cytoplasm is strongly eosinophilic.

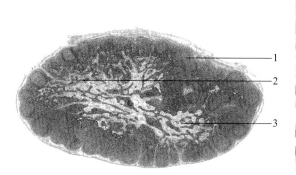

图 3-5a 淋巴结（100×）

Fig. 3-5a Lymph node (100×)

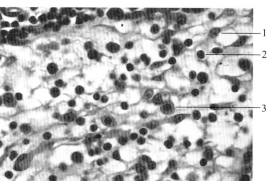

图 3-5b 淋巴结（400×）

Fig. 3-5b Lymph node (400×)

【示教切片】
【Teaching Sections】

❻ 切片 6：成纤维细胞

材料与方法：兔肉芽组织，HE 染色。

高倍镜观察：图 3-6 显示肉芽组织。肉芽组织中含有大量成纤维细胞（1），呈星状多突或梭形，细胞核卵圆形，胞质弱嗜碱性。

6. Section 6: Fibroblast

Materials and methods: Rabbit granulation tissue, HE staining.

HPM: Figure 3-6 shows granulation tissue, which contains many fibroblasts (1) with ovoid nucleus and weakly basophilic cytoplasm. These cells are stellate or fusiform.

❼ 切片 7：规则致密结缔组织

材料与方法：兔肌腱，HE 染色。

低倍镜观察：图 3-7，肌腱内胶原纤维排列方向一致。

7. Section 7: Regular dense connective tissue

Materials and methods: Rabbit's tendon, HE staining.

LPM: In Figure 3-7, the collagen fibers are parallel to each other.

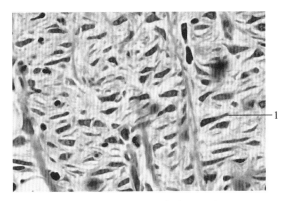

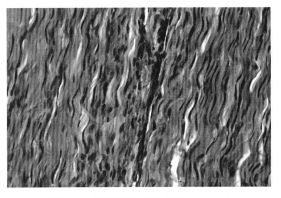

图 3-6 成纤维细胞（400×）

Fig. 3-6 Fibroblasts (400×)

图 3-7 规则致密结缔组织（200×）

Fig. 3-7 Regular dense connective tissue (200×)

⑧ 切片 8：浆细胞

材料与方法：人鼻息肉，HE 染色。

高倍镜观察：图 3-8 显示人鼻息肉，鼻息肉中大量的浆细胞（1）呈卵圆形，细胞核圆形或卵圆形，细胞质嗜碱性，核周围浅染。

8. Section 8: Plasma cells

Materials and methods: Human nasal polyps, HE staining.

HPM: Figure 3-8 shows human nasal polyp, which contains many ovoid plasma cells (1) with round and ovoid nucleus and basophilic cytoplasm. There is a light stained area in the periphery of nucleus, so-called halo.

⑨ 切片 9：网状纤维

材料与方法：人淋巴结，镀银法染色。

低倍镜观察：图 3-9 显示人淋巴结的网状纤维，网状纤维呈棕黑色，故又称嗜银纤维，交织成网状，构成淋巴结的支架。

9. Section 9: Reticular fibers

Materials and methods: Human lymph node, silver staining.

LPM: Figure 3-9 shows the reticular fibrils in lymph node. The reticular fibers are brown and

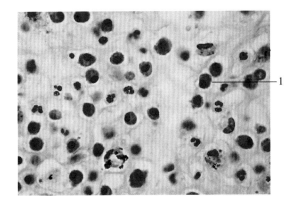

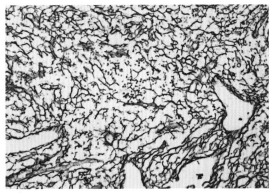

图 3-8 浆细胞（400×）

Fig. 3-8 Plasma cells (400×)

图 3-9 网状纤维（100×）

Fig. 3-9 Reticular fibers (100×)

called argentophil fibers, which are interwoven into nets, forming scaffolds of the lymph node.

【作业】

绘图并标注疏松结缔组织肠系膜铺片中的细胞和纤维。

【 Assignment 】

Drawing to describe the cells and fibers of loose connective tissue in stretched preparation of mesentery.

【思考题】

1. 试述浆细胞的光电镜结构特点。
2. 比较成纤维细胞和纤维细胞的光电镜结构特点。

【 Questions 】

1. Try to describe the morphologic characteristics of plasma cells.
2. To compare the morphologic characteristics of fibroblasts with fibrous cells.

【临床与科研联系英文阅读材料】 【 English Reading Material for Correlations with Clinic and Scientific Research 】

Keloid scars are excessive hyperplasia of dermal dense connective tissue in response to skin injuries. The keloid often invades into normal tissue beyond the injuries. Besides an ugly appearance, it sometimes can result in local pruritus or inflammation. It was reported that several signaling pathways were involved in Keloid formation, such as transforming growth factor β_1 (TGF β_1), insulin-like growth factor-1 (IGF-1), mitogen-activated protein kinase (MAPK), and integrin pathways. Four SNPs changes (rs873549, rs940187, rs1511412 and rs8032158), were found to be associated with keloid scars. The fact that the incidence rate of this disease is 15 times higher in blacks than that in whites indicates that the genetic factors play a role in this disease. However, it was also found that the local gene mutation, such as the 4th, 5th, 6th exon mutations of p53 gene, may be an important factor during keloid scar formation. The exact reasons of this disease are complex and still unidentified.

（迟晓春）

第4章 软骨和骨

Chapter ④ Cartilage and Bone

【实习内容】Contents of Observation

切片　Sections

观察切片	Observation Sections
1. 透明软骨（气管）	1. Hyaline cartilage（trachea）
2. 干骨磨片	2. Compact bone in ground sections
3. 膜内成骨（婴儿顶骨）	3. Intramembranous bone formation（fetus parietal bone）
4. 长骨形成（婴儿指）	4. Growth and ossification of long bone（fetus finger）

【目的要求】

1. 掌握透明软骨的形态结构特点。
2. 掌握长骨的构成，重点掌握骨单位的结构和功能。
3. 了解扁骨和长骨的形成。

【Objective】

1. To master the morphological characteristics of hyaline cartilage.

2. To master the structure of long bone, especially the structure and function of Haversian system.

3. To understand the formations of the flat bone and long bone.

【观察切片】
【Observation Sections】

❶ 切片 1：透明软骨

材料与方法：人气管，HE 染色。

低倍镜观察：图 4-1a 为气管的横断面，透明软骨位于气管的外膜，呈 "C" 形。透明软骨周围是软骨膜（1）。靠近软骨膜的软骨细胞（2）较为幼稚，体积小，扁椭圆形，单个散在分布。软骨中间的软骨细胞成群分布，每群由 2～8 个细胞构成，为同源细胞群（3）。

1. Section 1: Hyaline cartilage

Materials and methods: Human trachea, HE staining.

LPM: Figure 4-1a shows the cross section of trachea. The hyaline cartilage is found surrounding the trachea in a shape like letter C. The perichondrium (1) is localized at the surface of the hyaline cartilage. The chondrocytes (2) near the perichondriumare precursor cells with elliptic nuclei and are distributed as single cells. The chondrocytes in the middle of the cartilage appear in groups of 2-8 cells originating from a single chondrocyte. These groups are called isogenous aggregates (3).

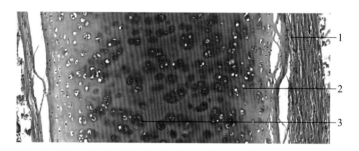

图 4-1a　透明软骨（40×）

Fig. 4-1a　Hyaline cartilage (40×)

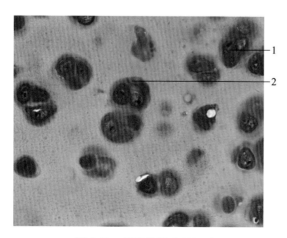

图 4-1b　透明软骨（400×）

Fig. 4-1b　Hyaline cartilage (400×)

高倍镜观察：图 4-1b，显示了透明软骨内部的软骨细胞（1）。细胞一般呈卵圆形，细胞呈弱嗜碱性。围绕软骨细胞的软骨基质含有较多的硫酸软骨素，有很强的嗜碱性，呈环形包绕软骨细胞，称为软骨囊（2）。

HPM: Figure 4-1b shows the morphology of the chondrocytes (1) in the center of the tissue. The chondrocytes are oval and weak basophilic. The cartilage matrix around the chondrocyte contains abundant chondroitin sulfate and has a strong basophilic property. It surrounds the chondrocyte in a circular shape and is called lacunae (2).

❷ 切片 2：干骨磨片

材料与方法：人股骨磨片，大力紫填染。

低倍镜观察：图 4-2a 为人股骨横断面。可见外环骨板、内环骨板和间骨板以及哈弗斯系统。哈弗斯系统由中间的哈弗斯管（1）和周围的哈弗斯骨板（2）构成。福克曼管（3）连接相邻哈弗斯管。在哈弗斯系统之间，可见呈半环形或者不规则的间骨板（4）。

图 4-2b 显示环骨板（1）围绕哈弗斯管（2）成同心圆状排列。相邻两层骨陷窝之间有骨小管（3）相连，骨小管围绕哈弗斯管呈放射状分布。哈弗斯系统的最外层有未着色区域，是黏合线（4）。

2. Section 2: Compact bone in transverse ground sections.

Materials and methods: Human femur, purple dye filling.

LPM: Figure 4-2a shows a cross section of human femur bone, which contains the outer circumferential lamella, inner circumferential lamella, intermediate lamella and Haversian system. Haversian system consists of central Haversian canal (1) and the peripheric Haversian lamella (2). Volkmann canal (3) connects the neighboring Haversian canals. There are several half circle or irregular shaped groups of parallel lamellae called interstitial lamella between the Haversian system (4).

Figure 4-2b shows that bone lacuna (1) around Haversain canal (2) distributes in circles. There are many bone canaliculi (3) radiating from the peripheric Haversian system between neighboring circles. There is an area called cement line (4) around a Haversian system, lacking of any canals or canaliculi and was unstained.

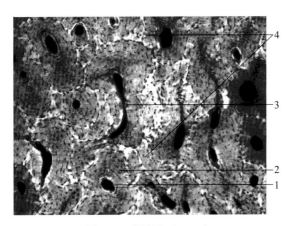

图 4-2a　骨磨片（40×）

Fig. 4-2a　Ground compact bone in transverse section (40×)

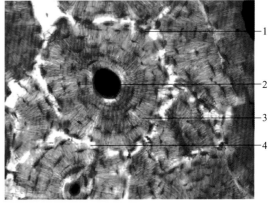

图 4-2b　骨单位（100×）

Fig. 4-2b　Osteon (100×)

❸ 切片 3：膜内成骨

材料与方法：胎儿顶骨，HE 染色。

低倍镜观察：图 4-3a 为胎儿顶骨切片。骨膜（1）为致密结缔组织，分布在骨组织两侧。新生骨片（2）为粉红色的扁形骨片，呈嗜酸性。骨组织表面成骨一侧分布有成骨细胞（3），为上皮样排列的成骨细胞。对侧骨组织表面分布有破骨细胞（4）。

高倍镜观察：图 4-3b，图 4-3c 为高倍镜照片。图 4-3b 为成骨细胞（1），细胞呈低柱状或扁平形，胞质嗜碱性。图 4-3c 为破骨细胞（2），为多核大细胞，胞质嗜酸性。

3. Section 3: Intramembranous ossification

Materials and methods: Parietal bone of fetus, HE staining.

LPM: Figure 4-3a shows parietal bone of infant. The bone membrane (1) consists of dense connective tissue and lies on both sides of the bone tissue. Newly formed parietal bone (2) is acidophilic, flat and pink. The osteoblasts (3) are always arranged in epitheliod array in the bone formation area. The osteoclasts (4) distribute in the opposite side of bone formation area.

HPM: The right two Figures 4-3 are osteoblasts (1) (Figure 4-3b) and osteoclasts (2) (Figure 4-3c) in high power magnification. The osteoblast is basophilic and is flat or short columnar cells. The osteoclast is large cell with multiple nuclei and acidophilic cytoplasm.

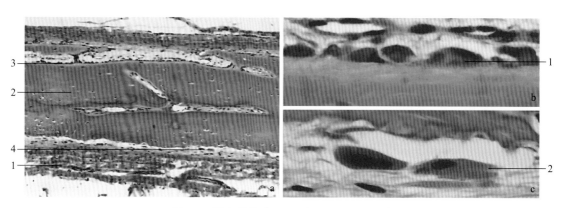

图 4-3　膜内成骨（a：40×；b，c：400×）

Fig. 4-3　Intramembranous bone formation (a: 40×, b, c: 400×)

❹ 切片 4：长骨形成

材料与方法：婴儿指，HE 染色。

低倍镜观察：图 4-4a-A 和图 4-4b 为婴儿手指切片。找到关节面（1），从关节面向骨髓腔（2）方向依次观察软骨贮备区、软骨增生区、软骨钙化区和成骨区。

高倍镜观察：图 4-4a-B、C、D、E 和图 4-4b 显示。在软骨贮备区（图 4-4a-B），软骨细胞体积小，散在分布，处于静止状态。在软骨增生区（图 4-4a-C），细胞分裂成同源细胞群，细胞纵行柱状排列，呈铜钱串状。在软骨钙化区（图 4-4a-D），软骨细胞肥大并呈空泡状，细胞退化、死亡。在成骨区（图 4-4a-E），在钙化的软骨基质外出现嗜酸性的新生骨片。在成骨区（图 4-4b），有破骨细胞（1）在溶骨。

4. Section 4: Growth and ossification of long bones

Materials and methods: Infant finger, HE staining.

LPM: Figure 4-4a-A and Figure 4-4b show sections of an infant finger. There is the resting zone, proliferative zone, calcified cartilage and ossification zone in an order from the articular surface (1) to the marrow cavity (2).

HPM: In Figure 4-4a-B, C, D, E and Figure 4-4b, cartilage cells in the resting zone (Figure 4-4a-B) remain quiescent and flat or rounded. In the proliferative zone (Figure 4-4a-C), the chondrocytes proliferate to isogenous aggregates in longitudinal columnar lining like copper coin. In the zone of calcified cartilage (Figure 4-4a-D), the chondrocytes become hypertrophic and vacuolated, a proceeding to cell retrogression or death. In the ossification zone (Figure 4-4a-E), new acidophilic bone tissue emerges in the calcified cartilage matrix. In the ossification zone (Figure 4-4b), osteoclasts (1) were dissolving bone.

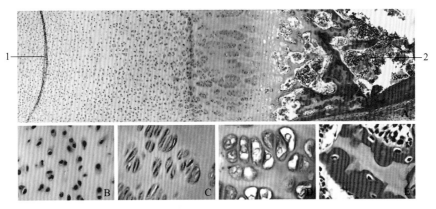

图 4-4a   长骨形成（低倍镜 40×，高倍镜 400×）

Fig. 4-4a   Growth and ossification of long bones (LPM 40×, HPM 400×)

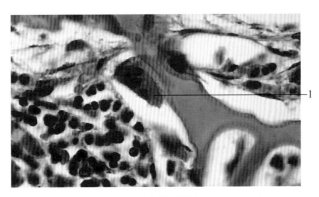

图 4-4b   成骨区中的破骨细胞（400×）

Fig. 4-4b   Osteoclast in the ossification zone (400×)

【作业】

绘图描述哈弗斯系统的组成。

【Assignment】

Draw and describe morphologic structures of the Haversian system.

【思考题】

1. 间骨板是如何形成的?
2. 你认为软骨囊和软骨陷窝是同一结构吗?

【Questions】

1. How interstitial lamella were formed?

2. Do you think cartilage capsule and cartilage lacuna are the same structure?

【临床与科研联系英文阅读材料】
【English Reading Material for Correlations with Clinic and Scientific Research】

Fractures are one of the most common tissue injuries. They often result from direct or indirect violent injuries or chronic fatigue damages, which lead to the destruction of bone continuity. Indirect fracture healing would undergo four periods: hematoma formation, fibrocartilaginous callus formation, bony callus formation, and bone remodeling. However, appropriate clinical treatment, with an anatomical reduction and rigid stablization, to prevent any gap formation, direct healing will happen and not necessarily go through all the four periods above. Bone lamella and/or Haversian systems will be regenerated much faster and reduce the healing time. Moreover, unlike other connective tissues, as we have known, bone is one of few tissues that can heal without forming a fibrous scar in either direct or indirect fracture healing.

（迟晓春）

第5章 血液和血细胞发生

Chapter 5 Blood and Hematopoiesis

【实习内容】Contents of Observation

标本　Sections

观察切片	Observation section
1. 血涂片	1. Blood smear
示教切片	**Teaching sections**
2. 网织红细胞	2. Reticulocytes
3. 骨髓涂片	3. Bone marrow smear

【目的要求】

1. 掌握成熟的血细胞的形态特点。
2. 了解网织红细胞。
3. 了解红系和粒系发生不同阶段的形态特点。

【Objective】

1. To master morphological features of mature blood cells.

2. To understand reticulocytes.

3. To understand morphological characteristics of different stages of erythropoiesis and granulopiesis.

【观察标本】
【Observation Section】

❶ 切片 1：血涂片

材料与方法：人血涂片，瑞氏染色。

高倍镜观察：

（1）红细胞：双凹圆盘形，胞质边缘染色深、中央染色浅，无细胞核。

（2）白细胞

① 中性粒细胞：图 5-1a 显示中性粒细胞，直径在 12～15μm 之间。胞质浅粉红色，含许多细小颗粒。细胞核可见两种形态：杆状核（A）和分叶核（B）。

② 嗜酸性粒细胞：图 5-1b 显示嗜酸性粒细胞，大小类似中性粒细胞。细胞质内充满粗大的嗜酸性颗粒，细胞核常分为两叶。

③ 嗜碱性粒细胞：图 5-1c 显示嗜碱性粒细胞，直径在 12～15μm 之间。细胞质内含有大量嗜碱性颗粒，可覆盖在核上，使细胞核不易分辨。

④ 淋巴细胞：图 5-1d 显示淋巴细胞，细胞核圆形或椭圆形，染色质致密，核染色深，胞质嗜碱性。根据直径分为大、中、小三型。一些淋巴细胞内含有较多嗜天青颗粒。

⑤ 单核细胞：图 5-1e 显示单核细胞，体积大，细胞直径在 12～20μm，细胞核偏离中心，形态多样，常见有肾形（A）、马蹄形（B）、不规则型（C）。胞质丰富，染色浅，嗜碱性，染为灰蓝色，内有嗜天青颗粒。

（3）血小板：图 5-1f 显示血小板，是不规则的细胞质小体，常成群分布在血细胞之间。中央为颗粒区，染色较深，周边染色浅，为透明区。

1. Section 1: Blood smear

Materials and methods: Human blood smear, Wright's staining.

HPM:

(1) Erythrocytes: Erythrocytes are biconcave disks, deep stained at the rim and light stained in the center, lacking of nucleus.

(2) Leukocytes

① Neutrophils: Figure 5-1a shows neutrophil. Neutrophils are about 12-15μm in diameter, with pink cytoplasm that contains numerous granules. The nucleus is rod (A) or segmented (B).

② Eosinophils: Figure 5-1b shows eosinophil. The cells typically have bilobed nuclei. The main identifying character is the abundance of large, red specific granules that are stained by eosin.

③ Basophils: Figure 5-1c shows basophil. Basophils are about 12-15μm in diameter. The nucleus is divided into two or more irregular lobes, but the large basophilic granules overlaying the nucleus obscure its shape.

④ Lymphocytes: Figure 5-1d shows lymphocytes. The lymphocytes constitute a family of leukocytes with spherical or ovoid nuclei, often indented, and condensed, with basophilic chromatin. Lymphocytes can be divided into small, medium and large lymphocytes according to their diameter. Some contain small azurophilic granules.

⑤ Monocytes: Figure 5-1e shows monocytes. Monocytes are large cells with diameter varying

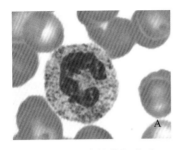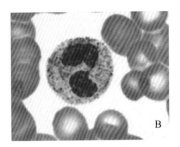

图 5-1a 中性粒细胞（1000×）（A：杆状核；B：分叶核）

Fig. 5-1a Neutrophil (1000×)(A: Rod-shaped nucleus, B: Segmented nucleus)

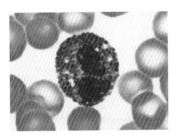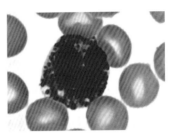

图 5-1b 嗜酸性粒细胞（1000×）　图 5-1c 嗜碱性粒细胞（1000×）

Fig. 5-1b Eosinophil (1000×)　Fig. 5-1c Basophil (1000×)

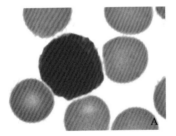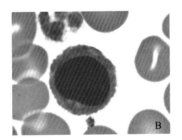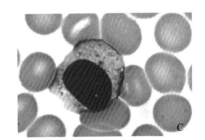

图 5-1d 淋巴细胞（1000×）（A：小淋巴细胞；B：中淋巴细胞；C：大淋巴细胞）

Fig. 5-1d Lymphocyte (1000×)(A: Small lymphocyte; B: Medium lymphocyte; C: Large lymphocyte)

from 12-20μm. The nucleus is large, off-center, and may be oval, kidney-shaped (A), horseshoe-shaped (B) or irregular (C). The nucleus stained lighter than that of large lymphocytes. The cytoplasm is basophilic and contains small azurophilic granules. These granules are distributed in the cytoplasm, giving rise to a bluish-gray color.

(3) Platelet: Figure 5-1f shows platelets. Platelets originate by cytoplasmic fragmentation, and often appear in clumps. Each platelet has a lightly stained peripheral zone and a central zone containing darker stained granules.

【示教切片】
【Teaching Sections】

❷ 切片 2：网织红细胞

材料与方法：小鼠血，煌焦油蓝染色。

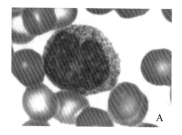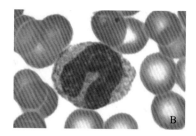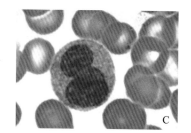

图 5-1e　单核细胞（1000×）

Fig. 5-1e　Monocyte (1000×)

高倍镜观察：图 5-2 显示网织红细胞（箭头），内有染为蓝色的细网状颗粒结构。

2. Section 2: Reticulocyte

Materials and methods: Mouse blood, brilliant cresyl blue staining.

HPM: Figure 5-2 shows reticulocytes (arrow). Reticulocytes contain fine reticulated granular structures, which are stained blue.

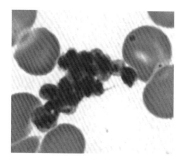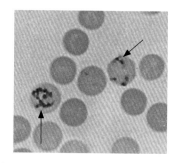

图 5-1f　血小板（1000×）　　　图 5-2　网织红细胞（箭头）（1000×）

Fig. 5-1f　Platelet (1000×)　　　Fig. 5-2　Reticulocyte (arrows)(1000×)

❸ 切片 3：骨髓涂片

材料与方法：人骨髓涂片，瑞氏染色。

高倍镜观察：

（1）红细胞系：包括原红细胞（图 5-3a）、早幼红细胞（图 5-3b）、中幼红细胞（图 5-3c）以及晚幼红细胞（图 5-3d）。

（2）粒细胞系：包括原粒细胞（图 5-3e）、早幼粒细胞（图 5-3f）、中幼粒细胞（图 5-3g）以及晚幼粒细胞（图 5-3h）。

3. Section 3: Bone marrow smear

Materials and methods: Human bone marrow smear, Wright's staining.

HPM:

(1) Erythropoiesis: Erythropoiesis includes proerythroblast (Figure 5-3a), basophilic erythroblast (Figure 5-3b), polychromatic erythroblast (Figure 5-3c), orthochromatic normoblast (Figure 5-3d).

(2) Granulopoiesis: Granulopoiesis includes myeloblast (Figure 5-3e), promyelocyte (Figure 5-3f), myelocyte (Figure 5-3g), metamyelocyte (Figure 5-3h).

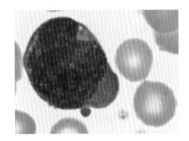

图 5-3a　原红细胞（1000×）

Fig. 5-3a　Proerythroblast
(1000×)

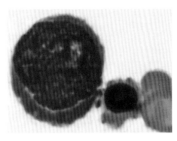

图 5-3b　早幼红细胞（1000×）

Fig. 5-3b　Basophilic erythroblast
(1000×)

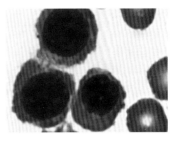

图 5-3c　中幼红细胞（1000×）

Fig. 5-3c　Polychromatic
erythroblast (1000×)

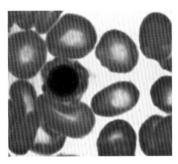

图 5-3d　晚幼红细胞（1000×）

Fig. 5-3d　Normoblast (1000×)

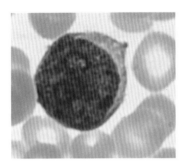

图 5-3e　原粒细胞（1000×）

Fig. 5-3e　Myeloblast (1000×)

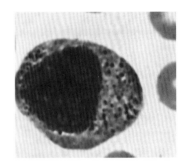

图 5-3f　早幼粒细胞（1000×）

Fig. 5-3f　Promyelocyte (1000×)

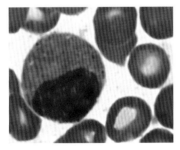

图 5-3g　中幼粒细胞（1000×）

Fig. 5-3g　Myelocyte (1000×)

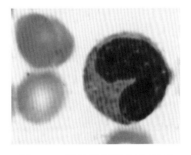

图 5-3h　晚幼粒细胞（1000×）

Fig. 5-3h　Metamyelocyte (1000×)

【思考题】

试述中性粒细胞的结构特点及功能。

【Question】

Try to describe the structure and function of neutrophils.

【临床与科研联系英文阅读材料】
【English Reading Material for Correlations with Clinic and Scientific Research】

Basophilia, an elevated basophil count in peripheral blood, rarely occurs in benign conditions. Mild basophilia may be part of a general inflammatory response to some infections, for example, smallpox, or influenza. It also occurs in allergic disorders or autoimmune inflammation such as rheumatoid arthritis or ulcerative colitis. More often, and for unclear reasons, basophilia is noted in malignant hematologic conditions called myeloproliferative disorders.

（舒丹毅）

第6章 肌组织

Chapter 6 Muscle Tissue

【实习内容】Contents of Observation

切片　Sections

观察切片	Observation Sections
1. 骨骼肌	1. Skeletal muscle
2. 心肌	2. Myocardium
3. 心肌闰盘（铁苏木精染色）	3. Intercalated disk（iron hematoxylin staining）
4. 平滑肌	4. Smooth muscle
示教切片	Teaching Sections
5. 骨骼肌（铁苏木精染色）	5. Skeletal muscle（iron hematoxylin staining）
6. 骨骼肌肌原纤维（电镜）	6. Myofibril of skeletal muscle（EM）
7. 心肌（电镜）	7. Myocardium（EM）

【目的要求】

1. 掌握骨骼肌、心肌、平滑肌的光镜形态结构特点及相互区别。
2. 区别骨骼肌与心肌的超微结构特点。
3. 掌握心肌闰盘结构，熟悉闰盘相接处的细胞连接类型。

【Objective】

1. To master the different morphological features among skeletal, cardiac and smooth muscles under light microscopy (LM).

2. To distinguish the ultrastructure of skeletal and cardiac muscles.

3. To master the structure of cardiac intercalated disk and to familiarize with the types of cell junction at the intercalated disk.

【观察切片】
【Observation Sections】

❶ 切片 1：骨骼肌

材料与方法：兔骨骼肌，HE 染色。

（1）骨骼肌纵断面

低倍镜观察：图 6-1a 显示骨骼肌纵断面纤维呈细长条形，细胞核在骨骼肌纤维周边肌膜下，每个肌纤维有多个细胞核。细胞核呈椭圆或细长形。肌纤维间的结缔组织内可见小血管（1）。

高倍镜观察：图片 6-1b 显示骨骼肌纤维纵行排列。细胞核（1）位于肌膜下，细胞质内由暗带和明带构成了明暗相间的横纹（2）。肌纤维间有少量的结缔组织，结缔组织内可见成纤维细胞。

Materials and methods: Rabbit skeletal muscle, HE staining.

(1) Longitudinal section of skeletal muscle

LPM: Figure 6-1a shows the skeletal muscle fibers as elongated and cylindrical cells. They are multinucleated. The nuclei are oval or elongated, basophilic, and located at the periphery of the cell. Small blood vessels (1) are seen in the connective tissue between muscle fibers.

HPM: Figure 6-1b shows the skeletal muscle in longitudinal arrangement. The nucleus (1) is under the sarcolemma of each cell. The cytoplasm is characterized by cross-striations (2) that consist of alternating dark bands and light bands. Between muscle fibers there are little connective tissues, which contain scattered fibroblasts.

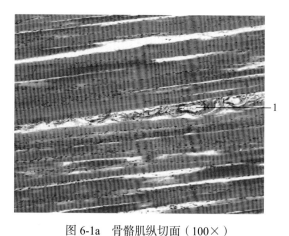

图 6-1a 骨骼肌纵切面（100×）

Fig. 6-1a Longitudinal section of skeletal muscle (100×)

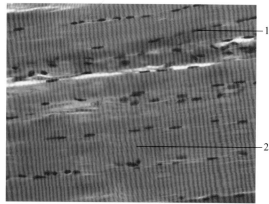

图 6-1b 骨骼肌纵切面（400×）

Fig. 6-1b Longitudinal section of skeletal muscle (400×)

（2）骨骼肌横断面

低倍镜观察：图片 6-1c 显示骨骼肌的结构组成。包绕在整块肌肉外面的结缔组织为肌外膜（未显示），每一肌束外面的薄层结缔组织为肌束膜（1）。每条肌纤维周围为肌内膜（2）。

每个肌纤维的细胞膜称作肌膜。在结缔组织间可见血管（3）、神经（4）通过。

高倍镜观察：图片 6-1d 显示骨骼肌呈多边形或圆形，细胞核（1）位于肌膜下，肌浆内隐约可见的点状结构为肌原纤维（2）的横断面。

(2) Transverse section of skeletal muscle

LPM: Figure 6-1c shows the structure of skeletal muscle. The epimysium (not shown) surrounds the whole muscle externally. The perimysium (1) subdivides the muscle internally into fascicles. The endomysium (2) surrounds individual muscle fibers. The membrane of each muscle fiber is called sarcolemma. The blood vessels (3) and nerves (4) can be observed in connective tissues.

HPM: Figure 6-1d shows skeletal muscle fiber in round to polygonal shape. The nuclei (1) are under the sarcolemma. The sarcoplasm of each fiber looks punctate because of tightly packed myofibrils (2).

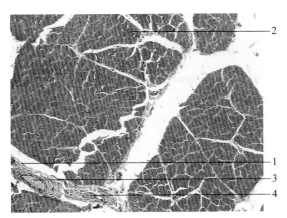
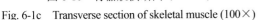
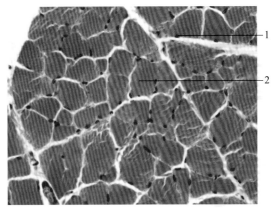

图 6-1c　骨骼肌横断面（100×）

Fig. 6-1c　Transverse section of skeletal muscle (100×)

图 6-1d　骨骼肌横断面（400×）

Fig. 6-1d　Transverse section of skeletal muscle (400×)

❷ 切片 2：心肌

材料与方法：人心肌，HE 染色。

低倍镜观察：图 6-2a 显示心肌纤维的纵断面呈短柱状，有分支。有的切面呈斜断面。细胞核（1）在细胞的中央。心肌纤维的横断面（图 6-2b）呈圆形、椭圆形，核（1）在中央。心肌纤维间可见毛细血管（2）和结缔组织（3）。

2. Section 2: Myocardium

Materials and methods: Human myocardium, HE staining.

Under LPM, Figure 6-2a shows the cardiac muscle cells cut in longitudinal section. The cardiac muscle cell is short column-shape, with branches. Some sections show as oblique sections. The nucleus (1) is located in the center of the cell. The cross section of cardiac fiber (Figure 6-2b) is round, ovoid shapes, with central nucleus (1). Micro-vessel (2) and loose connective tissue (3) can be observed between cardiac fibers.

高倍镜观察：图 6-2c 显示纵断面的心肌纤维呈短柱分枝状。细胞核（1）位于肌纤维中央，有时可见双核（2），细胞核两端肌浆丰富，有时可见脂褐素颗粒。心肌细胞相邻处可见阶梯状、直板状线样结构，为心肌闰盘（3），染色深，往往与心肌细胞长轴垂直。图 6-2d 显

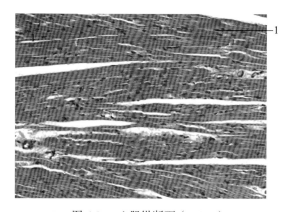

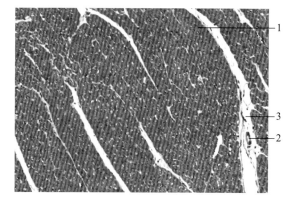

图 6-2a　心肌纵断面（100×）

Fig. 6-2a　Longitudinal section of cardiac muscle (100×)

图 6-2b　心肌横断面（100×）

Fig. 6-2b　Transverse section of cardiac muscle (100×)

示横断面的心肌细胞，核（1）位于中央。每个心肌细胞周围由基膜和网状纤维组成的肌内膜包绕。肌内膜中可见成纤维细胞的细胞核（2）和毛细血管。

Under HPM, Figure 6-2c shows longitudinal section of cardiac fiber. Each cell has an eosinophilic sarcoplasm surrounding a single, centrally placed, ovoid nucleus, but occasional binucleated (2) cells are seen. The Lipofuscin can be accumulated in the cytoplasm. Intercalated discs (3) of cardiac muscle cells can be observed in the cell junctions, where cells and their branches meet. The discs have the appearance of steps in staircase, or in linear shapes, deep-staining, perpendicular to the long axis of the cell. Figure 6-2d shows the cross section of cardiac muscle cells. The nuclei (1) occupy the center of cells. Each cardiac muscle cell is surrounded by basal lamina and endomysium, where fibroblast nuclei (2) and capillary can be observed.

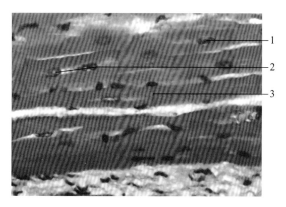

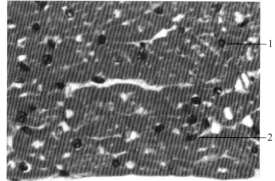

图 6-2c　心肌纵断面（400×）

Fig. 6-2c　Longitudinal section of cardiac muscle (400×)

图 6-2d　心肌横断面（400×）

Fig. 6-2d　Transverse Section of cardiac muscle (400×)

❸ 切片 3：心肌闰盘

材料与方法：人心肌、铁苏木精染色。

高倍镜观察：图 6-3 显示心肌细胞间呈直线或阶梯状方式嵌合的连接方式，即闰盘结构（1）。图片中可见细胞核位于肌纤维中央（2），部分心肌细胞可见双核（3），细胞质内隐约可见脂褐素（4）。心肌纤维间可见结缔组织、毛细血管（5）及成纤维细胞（6）。

3. Section 3: Myocardial intercalated disc

Materials and methods: Human cardiac muscle, iron hematoxylin staining.

HPM: The Figure 6-3 shows the intercalated disc (1), which connects adjacent cells in an eosinophilic straight line or stair-step pattern. The nucleus is visible in the center of the muscle fiber (2). There are double nuclei (3) in some cells. The lipofuscin (4) also can be observed faintly. Connective tissue and capillaries (5), fibroblasts (6) are seen among myocardial fibers.

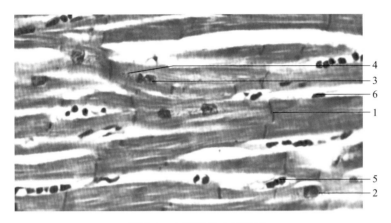

图 6-3　心肌闰盘（400×）

Fig. 6-3　intercalated discs of myocardium (400×)

❹ 切片 4：平滑肌（膀胱壁）

材料与方法：兔的膀胱，HE 染色。

低倍镜观察：图 6-4a 显示在膀胱变移上皮下方可见平滑肌结构，其中部分结构显示为平滑肌纵切面（1），部分结构显示为平滑肌横切面（2）。

高倍镜观察：图 6-4b 上显示长梭形的平滑肌细胞呈细胞质嗜酸性，均质无横纹。细胞核（1）位于中央，长杆状、嗜碱性。肌纤维间可见成纤维细胞（2）。图 6-4b 下显示横断面平滑

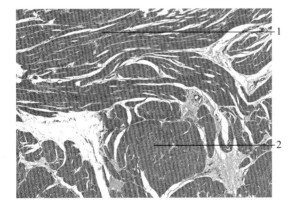

图 6-4a　平滑肌（100×）

Fig. 6-4a　Smooth muscle (100×)

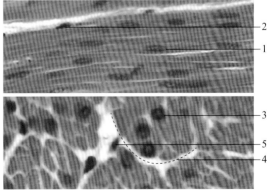

图 6-4b　平滑肌纵 / 横切面（400×）

Fig. 6-4b　Longitudinal/ Transverse section of smooth muscle (400×)

肌纤维，细胞核（3）位于中央。肌纤维之间可见肌束膜（4），内可见成纤维细胞（5）。

4. Section 4: Smooth muscle (urinary bladder wall)

Materials and methods: Rabbit, urinary bladder, paraffin-embedded, HE staining.

LPM: Figure 6-4a shows that smooth muscle structure was seen below the transitional epithelium of the bladder. Some of the structures are shown as longitudinal sections of smooth muscle (1), and some of them are shown as smooth muscle cross-sections (2).

HPM: Figure 6-4b-upper shows that smooth muscle cell has an eosinophilic cytoplasm, which is homogeneous and unstriated. The nucleus is located at the cell center, long rod-shape and basophilic. Between the fibers there are fibroblasts (2). Figure 6-4b-lower shows the transverse-section of smooth muscle. The nucleus (3) is located at the cell center. The endomysium (4) is seen among the fibers, in which the fibroblast (5) can be observed.

【示教切片】
【Teaching Sections】

⑤ 切片 5: 骨骼肌（铁苏木精染色）

材料与方法：人骨骼肌，铁苏木精染色。

高倍镜观察：图 6-5a 显示骨骼肌纤维纵行排列，肌纤维显示出明暗相间的横纹（1），细胞多核，细胞核（2）位于肌膜下。肌纤维间有少量的结缔组织，结缔组织内可见成纤维细胞（3）。图 6-5b 显示骨骼肌横切面，细胞核（1）位于细胞周边肌膜下。肌束膜结缔组织处（2）可见成纤维细胞（3）和毛细血管（4）。

5. Section5: Skeletal muscle (Iron hematoxylin staining)

Materials and methods: Human skeletal muscle, iron hematoxylin staining.

HPM: Figure 6-5a shows the longitudinally arranged skeletal muscle fibers with regular cross-striations (1). They are multinucleated. The nuclei (2) are located at peripheral positions in the cell. Among muscle fibers there are little connective tissues, which contains nuclei of scattered fibroblasts (3). Figure 6-5b shows the transverse section of skeletal muscle. The nuclei (1) are under

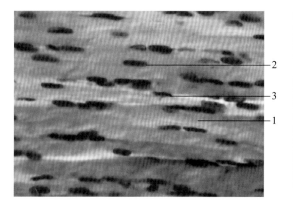

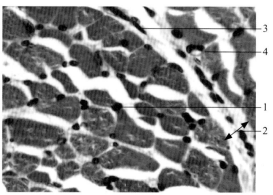

图 6-5a　骨骼肌纵切面（400×）

Fig. 6-5a　Longitudinal section of skeletal muscles (400×)

图 6-5b　骨骼肌横切面（400×）

Fig. 6-5b　Transverse section of skeletal muscles (400×)

the sarcolemma of each cell. In the connective tissue perimysium (2), there are fibroblasts (3) and capillaries (4).

⑥ 切片 6：骨骼肌（电镜）

材料与方法：小鼠骨骼肌，电镜，10 000×。

电镜观察：图 6-6 显示骨骼肌细胞内平行排列的肌原纤维，肌原纤维（1）（图中虚线所示单个肌原纤维）与骨骼肌细胞长轴平行。肌原纤维的暗带 /A 带（2）与明带 /I 带（3）构成明暗相间的横纹。暗带由粗、细肌丝相互交叠而成，明带只有细肌丝组成。明带中央是 Z 线（4）。相邻两条 Z 线之间的一段肌原纤维为肌节（5）。

6. Section 6: Skeletal muscle (EM)

Materials and methods: Mouse, skeletal muscle, EM, 10 000x

EM: Figure 6-6 shows that the skeletal muscle cells are composed of parallel-arranged myofibrils (1) are parallel to the long axis of skeletal muscle cells. The dark bands/A bands (2), and light bands/I bands (3) of myofibril form the cross-striation. The A band consists of both thick and thin myofilaments that overlap. The I band consists of only thin myofilament. The Z disk (4) is located at the center of light band. The segment between two Z disks forms a sarcomere (5).

⑦ 切片 7：浦肯野纤维

材料与方法：小鼠心壁，HE 染色。

低倍镜观察：图 6-7，心肌浦肯野纤维（1）也称束细胞，是一种特殊的心肌纤维，分布于心室的心内膜（2）下层。比普通的心肌细胞（3）直径大，肌浆多，着色浅，核在细胞中心。

7. Section 7: Myocardial Purkenje cells

Materials and methods: Mouse myocardium, HE staining.

LPM: Figuer 6-7, the myocardial Purkenje cells (1) also are called cardiac bundle cells, which are specialized myocardial fibers and located under the ventrical endocardium (2). Purkinje fibers are larger and paler than ordinary myocytes (3), with the nucleus at the center.

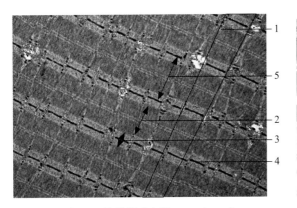

图 6-6　骨骼肌（电镜，10 000×）

Fig. 6-6　Skeletal muscle (EM, 10 000×)

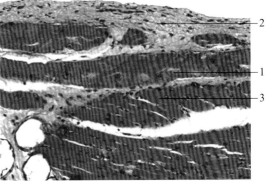

图 6-7　心肌浦肯野细胞

Fig. 6-7　Cardiac Purkinje cells

⑧ 切片 8：心肌（电镜）

材料与方法：小鼠心肌，电镜，10 000×。

电镜观察：图 6-8a 显示心肌细胞内平行排列的肌原纤维（1），细胞核（2）位于心肌细胞中央。线粒体（3）线性排列于肌纤维之间。肌原纤维同样由暗带（4）和明带（5）构成横纹结构。明带中央可见 Z 线（6）。肌细胞之间可见成纤维细胞核（7）和结缔组织。图 6-8b 显示两个心肌细胞（A 和 B）之间的闰盘结构。在心肌的横向连接部位有中间连接（1）和桥粒（2）。在纵向连接的部位有缝隙连接。

8. Section 8. Cardiac muscle (EM)

Materials and methods: Mouse myocardia EM, 10 000×.

EM: Figure 6-8a shows that the cardiac muscle cells are composed of parallel-arranged myofibrils (1). The nucleus (2) is located at the center of the cardiac cell. The mitochondria (3) are arranged linearly among myofibrils, in which the dark bands (4) and light bands (5) form cross striation. Z disk (6) is located at the center of light band. The fibroblast (7) and connective tissue can be observed among muscle fibers. Figure 6-8b shows the myocardial intercalated disc between two cardiac cells (A and B). There are fascia adherens (1) and a desmosome (2) in the transverse junction of cardiac cells, but a gap junction in the lateral portion of an intercalated disc.

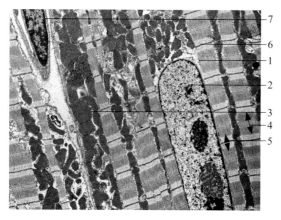

图 6-8a　心肌（电镜，10 000×）
Fig. 6-8a　Cardiac muscle (EM, 10 000×)

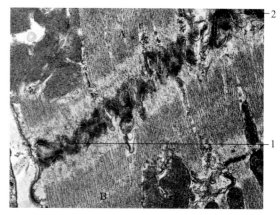

图 6-8b　闰盘（电镜，25 000×）
Fig. 6-8b　Intercalated disc (EM, 25 000×)

【思考题】

1. 比较光镜下骨骼肌、心肌、平滑肌组织结构的异同点。
2. 骨骼肌、心肌纤维出现横纹的结构基础是什么？
3. 试述骨骼肌纤维的收缩机制及其超微结构基础。
4. 心肌纤维的连接方式是什么？其功能是什么？

【Questions】

1. To compare the structural differences among skeletal, cardiac and smooth muscles.

2. What are the structural basis of striated bands of skeletal and cardiac muscles?

3. Try to describe the contraction mechanism of a skeletal muscle fiber and its ultrastructural basis.

4. What is the intercellular connection pattern of cardiac fibers? what is its function?

【临床与科研联系英文阅读材料】
【English Reading Material for Correlations with Clinic and Scientific Research】

Rigor Mortis is the stiffening of the body after death because of the loss of Adenosine Triphosphate (ATP) from the body's muscles. ATP is the substance that allows energy to flow to the muscles and help them work. Without ATP, the muscles become stiff and inflexible. Rigor normally appears within the body around two hours after the deceased has passed away with the facial and upper neck and shoulder muscles first to visibly suffer from its effects. This is because the facial muscles have contracted as ATP drains from them. Once the contracting of all the body's muscles has taken place the state of Rigor has achieved-technically referred to as the Rigid Stage—the process normally lasts from eight to twelve hours, after which time the body is completely stiff. This fixed state lasts approximately for another eighteen hours. In contrary to common perception, the process of Rigor Mortis actually does reverse and the body returns to a flaccid state; the muscles lose their tightness in the reverse of how they gain it. In other words, those larger muscles that contract last will lose their stiffness first and return to their pre-Rigor condition. Rigor Mortis is a good means of indicating time of death as it is normally visible within the first thirty-six to forty-eight hours after death; after that it leaves the body.

（王大亮　常智杰）

第 7 章 神 经 组 织

Chapter 7 Nervous Tissue

【实习内容】Contents of Observation

 切片　Sections

观察切片	Observation Sections
1. 多极神经元（脊髓）	1. Multipolar neuron（spinal code）
2. 浦肯野细胞（小脑）	2. Purkinje cell（cerebellum）
3. 有髓神经纤维（坐骨神经）	3. Myelinated nerve fibers（sciatic nerve）
4. 有髓神经纤维（银染）（坐骨神经）	4. Myelinated nerve fibers（silver staining）（sciatic nerve）
5. 触觉小体（皮肤）	5. Tactile corpuscle（skin）
6. 环层小体（皮肤）	6. Lamellar corpuscle（skin）
7. 运动终板（肌肉）	7. Motor end plate（muscle）
示教切片	Teaching Sections
8. 多极神经元（氯化金染）	8. Multipolar neuron（gold chloride staining）
9. 浦肯野细胞（银染）	9. Purkinje cell（silver staining）
10. 神经原纤维（氯化金染）	10. Neurofibril（gold chloride staining）
11. 尼氏体（硫堇 - 苦力紫）	11. Nissle body（thio-bitter violet）
12. 轴 - 树突触（电镜）	12. Axon-dendritic synapses（EM）

【目的要求】

1. 掌握多极神经元的形态及光镜结构特点。
2. 掌握小脑浦肯野细胞的位置、大小及形态结构特点。
3. 掌握周围有髓神经纤维的构造。
4. 了解神经末梢的种类及组织结构。
5. 熟悉突触的结构。

【Objective】

1. To master the morphological features of multipolar neuron under LM.
2. To master the localization, size and morphological structure of cerebellar Purkinje cells.
3. To master the structure of peripheral myelinated nerve fibers.
4. To understand the types and structures of nerve ending.
5. To be familiar with the structure of synapsis.

【观察切片】
【Observation Sections】

❶ 切片1：多极神经元

材料与方法：猫脊髓，HE 染色。

高倍镜观察：图 7-1 显示脊髓前角运动细胞（ ↘ ），内含细胞核（1）、明显的核仁（2）和大量的尼氏体（3），可观察到神经元的轴突（4）和树突（5）。轴突只有一个，自胞体伸出区域，不含尼氏体叫轴丘（6）。在 α- 运动神经元的周围，有较多的神经胶质细胞（7），体积较小，细胞突起不易观察。

1. Section 1: Multipolar neuron

Materials and methods: Cat spinal cord, HE staining.

HPM: Figure 7-1shows the spinal anterior horn motor neuron (↘), containing the nucleus (1), prominent nucleolus (2) and large amount of Nissl bodies (3). The α-motor neuron axons (4) and dendrites (5) can be distinguished. There is only one axon, which projects from soma and without Nissl substance in the region called Axis hillock (6). Around the α-motor neuron, there are a lot of neuroglia cells (7), which have small soma, and cellular processes not easily observed.

❷ 切片2：浦肯野细胞

材料与方法：小鼠小脑，HE 染色。

高倍镜观察：图 7-2 显示浦肯野细胞（ ↗ ）位于小脑的分子层（1）与颗粒层（2）之间，细胞胞体（3）较大，复杂的树突（4）延伸到小脑的分子层，轴突则延伸到颗粒层。

2. Section 2: Purkinje cell

Materials and methods: Cerebellum of mouse, HE staining.

HPM: Figure 7-2 shows that Purkinje cell (↗) is located between molecular layer (1) and

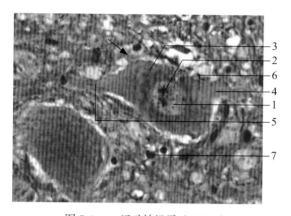

图 7-1 α- 运动神经元（400×）

Fig. 7-1 α-motor neuron（400×）

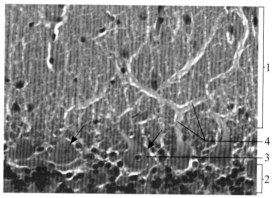

图 7-2 浦肯野细胞（400×）

Fig. 7-2 Purkinje cell（400×）

granular layer (2) in the cerebellum, with a large soma (3). The elaborated dendrites (4) extend into the molecular layer, and axon projects into the granular layer.

❸ 切片 3：有髓神经纤维（纵断面）

材料与方法：猫坐骨神经，HE 染色。

低倍镜观察：图 7-3a 显示神经纵断面上，可见许多平行排列的神经纤维。包围在整个神经外面，由致密结缔组织构成的结构为神经外膜（1），内含小血管和神经。坐骨神经被分成很多束，每个神经束的周围由结缔组织组成神经束膜（2），神经束由很多神经纤维组成，每根神经纤维周围的薄层结缔组织为神经内膜。

3. Section 3: Myelinated nerve fibers (longitudinal section)

Materials and methods: Sciatic nerve of the cat, HE staining.

LPM: Figure 7-3a shows a portion of a peripheral nerve cut in longitudinal section surrounded by a dense, connective tissue layer called the epineurium (1), which contains small blood vessels and nerves. The sciatic nerve is separated into bundles, which are surrounded by perineurium (2). The fascicles are composed of nerve fibers, which is surrounded by endoneurium.

高倍镜观察：图 7-3b 显示神经的纵断面。髓鞘（1）部分由于脂肪含量较高，经过石蜡包埋后溶解而成为空泡状。施万细胞核（2）狭长，椭圆形。施万细胞之间的狭窄处为郎飞结（3）。轴突（4）位于神经纤维的中间。

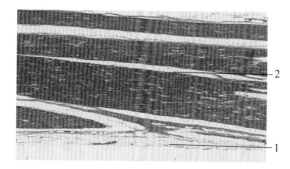

图 7-3a 周围神经（20×）

Fig. 7-3a Peripheral nerve（20×）

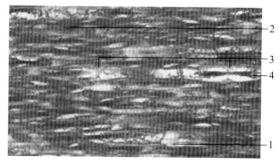

图 7-3b 周围神经（400×）

Fig. 7-3b Peripheral nerve（400×）

HPM: Figure 7-3b shows the peripheral nerve cut in longitudinal section. Myelin sheaths (1) appear vacuolated because of high lipid content with the effects of paraffin embedding on the tissue sample. Schwann cells (2) have elongated and oval nuclei. The narrow place at the junction between two contiguous Schwann cells is called Ranvier Node (3). The axon (4) is located at the center of nerve fiber.

❹ 切片 4：有髓神经纤维（银染）

材料与方法：猫坐骨神经，银染。

神经纵切面：图 7-4a 显示纵切的周围神经，可见许多呈波浪状平行排列的神经纤维（1），神经外膜包绕在整个神经外面（2）。

4. Section 4: Myelinared nerve fibers（silver staining）

Materials and methods: Sciatic nerve of the cat, silver staining

Nerve in longitudinal section: Figure 7-4a shows the longitudinal section of peripheral nerve (1) surrounded by the epineurium (2).

高倍镜：图 7-4b 显示神经束由很多神经纤维组成，通过银染法髓鞘溶解显示为透明区域（1），轴突呈浅棕色（2），施万细胞核（3）位于神经纤维周边。施万细胞间，轴突外无髓鞘包绕之处可见郎飞结（4）。

HPM: Figure 7-4b shows that the fascicle consists of nerve fibers. The myelin sheath (1) is stained black, and the axon is stained light brown (2) by silver staining. The nuclei of Schwann cells (3) are located in the peripheral nerve fiber and stain black. Ranvier Node (4) is located at the junction of Schwann cells, where the axon is not covered by myelins.

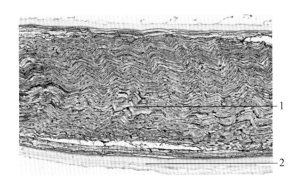 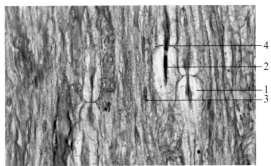

图 7-4a 神经纵断面（50×）　　　　　图 7-4b 神经纵断面（200×）

Fig. 7-4a Longitudinal section of a nerve (50×)　　Fig. 7-4b Longitudinal section of a nerve (200×)

神经横切面：图 7-4c 显示横切的周围神经，由神经外膜（1）包绕。神经外膜为不规则致密结缔组织，与神经束膜（2）相连续。神经束由神经纤维（3）组成。

Nerve in cross section: Figure 7-4c shows the transversal section of peripheral nerve surrounded by the epineurium (1), which is irregular dense connective tissue. The epineurium is continuous with perineurium (2). The Fascicle (3) consists of nerve fibers (4).

高倍镜：图 7-4d 显示神经束外面包绕神经束膜（1）。神经束由神经纤维（2）组成，每根神经纤维外面包绕神经内膜（3）。银染制片中髓鞘发生溶解，显示为透明区域，轴突（4）

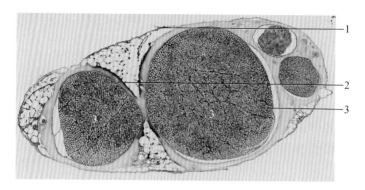

图 7-4c　神经横断面（40×）

Fig. 7-4c　Cross section of a nerve (40×)

染成棕色。

HPM: Figure 7-4d shows that the nerve bundle is surrounded by perineurium (1), composed of many nerve fibers (2). Each nerve fiber is surrounded by an endoneurium (3). The myelin sheath is disappeared in histological preparation using silver staining, and shows as a clear space. The axon (4) stains brown.

❺ 切片 5：触觉小体

材料与方法：人皮肤，HE 染色。

低倍镜观察：图 7-5 显示真皮的乳头内，可见椭圆形的触觉小体（1），其长轴与皮肤表面垂直，外周有结缔组织膜包裹。囊内的细胞（2）扁平排列，有髓神经纤维进入触觉小体时失去髓鞘，分支盘绕在扁平细胞之间。

5. Section 5: Tactile corpuscle

Materials and Methods: Skin of human, paraffin embedding, HE staining.

LPM: Figure 7-5 shows the oval tactile corpuscle (1) in the dermal papilla, whose long axis is perpendicular to the skin surface. It consists of flattened supportive cells (2) arranged as horizontal lamellae surrounded by a connective tissue capsule. The myelinated nerve fiber will lose its myelin sheath in Meissner's corpuscles, with its branches coiled among flat cells.

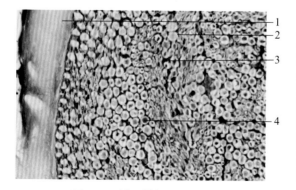

图 7-4d　神经横断面（200×）

Fig. 7-4d　Cross section of a nerve (200×)

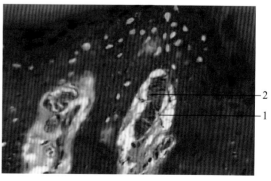

图 7-5　触觉小体（200×）

Fig. 7-5　Tactile corpuscle (200×)

❻ 切片 6：环层小体

材料与方法：人皮肤，HE 染色。

低倍镜观察：图 7-6 显示为皮肤真皮深层，可见两个卵圆形的环层小体结构（1），其被囊由数十层扁平细胞（2）呈同心圆排列组成，中轴为一均质性的圆柱体（3），有髓神经纤维失去髓鞘后穿行于柱内。环层小体感受压力和振动觉。

6. Section 6: Lamellar corpuscle

Materials and Methods: Skin of human, HE staining.

LPM: Figure 7-6 shows two oval lamellar corpuscles (1) in the deep layer of skin dermis. Its capsule consists of dozens of layers of concentric lamellated flattened cells (2). The center of the corpuscle is a homogeneous cylinder (3), which is a single afferent unmyelinated neurite at the receptive region. Lamellar corpuscles is responsible for sensitivity to vibration and pressure.

❼ 切片 7：运动终板

材料与方法：小鼠肌肉，氯化金法制作，压片。

低倍镜观察：图 7-7 显示为一块骨骼肌组织，由若干条骨骼肌纤维（1）组成，有髓神经纤维（2）末端发出若干分支，沿着肌细胞表面继续延伸，髓鞘消失，末端膨大附着于骨骼肌，纤维表面形成运动终板（3）。

7. Section 7: Motor end plate

Materials and methods: muscle of mouse, gold chloride staining, tissue compression.

LPM: Figure 7-7 shows skeletal muscle tissue composed of a number of skeletal muscle fibers (1). The myelinated nerve fibers (2) at the ends send out branches, which extend along the surface of the muscle cells, loss the myelin sheath, and the ends of the expansion attach to the skeletal muscle, to form the motor end plate (3).

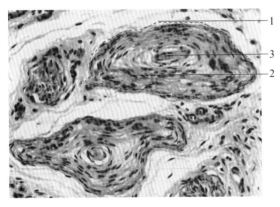

图 7-6　环层小体（100×）

Fig. 7-6　Lamellar corpuscle（100×）

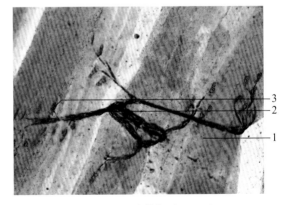

图 7-7　运动终板（100×）

Fig. 7-7　Motor end plate（100×）

【示教切片】
【Teaching Sections】

❽ 切片 8：多极神经元

材料与方法：猫脊髓，氯化金染色。

低倍镜观察：图 7-8 显示在脊髓灰质区可见胞体较大的 α- 运动神经元（1）为多极神经元，胞体内含细胞核（2）和明显的核仁（3），以及胞体发出的树突（4）。神经纤维显示为细黑线结构（5），其与 α- 运动神经元构成突触（6）。

8. Section 8: Multipolar neuron

Materials and methods: Spinal cord of the cat, Gold chloride staining.

LPM: Figure 7-8 show α-motor neuron with a larger body as a multipolar neuron (1) in the gray area of spinal cord. The perikaryon contains the nucleus (2), a prominent nucleolus (3), and dendrites (4) extended by the body. The nerve fibers (5) showed as black lines, form synapses (6) with dendrites of α-motor neuron.

❾ 切片 9：浦肯野细胞

材料与方法：人小脑，银染。

低倍镜观察：图 7-9 显示小脑分为分子层（M）、浦肯野细胞层（P）和颗粒层（G）。浦肯野细胞位于分子层和颗粒层之间，由胞体（1）、细胞核（2）和许多树突（3）组成，另外可见篮状细胞的轴突包绕浦肯野细胞的胞体构成的篮状网（4），分子层可见平行纤维（5），颗粒层可见大量颗粒细胞（6）等结构。

9. Section 9: Purkinje cells

Materials and methods: Cerebellum of human, silver staining.

LPM: Figure 7-9 shows that the cerebellum is separated into three layers, molecular (M), Purkinje cell (P), and granular layers (G). The Purkinje cells are located between the molecular and granular layers, consisting of the cell body (1), a nucleus (2) and a larger dendrite (3). The basket-like network of axons from basket (4) neurons surrounding the cell body of Purkinje, also can be observed. The dendritic tree extend into the cortex surface, deeper into molecular layer, and repeatedly branch. There are also axons of parallel fibers (5) in the molecular layer, granular cells (6) in the granular layer.

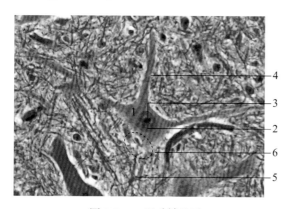

图 7-8　α- 运动神经元

Fig. 7-8　α-Motor neuron

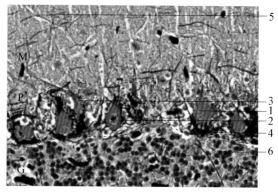

图 7-9　小脑浦肯野细胞

Fig. 7-9　Cerebellum Purkinje cell

❿ 切片 10：神经原纤维

材料与方法：猫脊髓，氯化金染色。

高倍镜观察：图 7-10 显示在神经元胞质内神经原纤维（1）交织成网状，银染切片中呈棕黑色细丝，伸入树突或是轴突。结构（2）示神经纤维。

10. Section10: Neurofibrils

Materials and methods: Spinal cord of the cat, gold chloride staining.

HPM: Figure 7-10 demonstrates the neurofibrils (1) in the neuronal cytoplasm, shown as black filaments by silver staining. The structure (2) shows the nerve fiber.

⑪ 切片 11：尼氏体

材料与方法：猫脊髓，硫堇 - 苦力紫染色。

高倍镜观察：图 7-11 显示在硫堇染色法下尼氏体（1）呈深蓝紫色颗粒或斑块状，细胞核（2）淡蓝色，而核仁（3）呈深蓝色。可见神经元的轴突（4）和树突（5）。星形胶质细胞（6）的细胞核略大，染色质稀疏，而少突胶质细胞（7）的细胞核小，染色质致密，常位于胞体或轴突附近。

11. Section 11: Nissl body

Materials and methods: Spinal cord of the cat, thio-bitter violet staining.

HPM: Figure 7-11 shows that the Nissl body (1) is dark blue granules or plaques in thionine staining. The nucleus (2) is stained as light-blue, but the nucleoli (3) are dark blue. The axon (4) and dendrites (5) can be distinguished. The astrocyte (6) has a larger, oval nucleus with light chromatin, but the oligodendrocyte (7) has a smaller nucleus with a dense chromatin pattern, which is always located near perikaryon or axon.

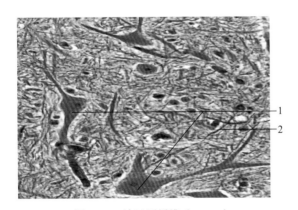

图 7-10　神经原纤维（400×）
Fig. 7-10　Neurofibrils（400×）

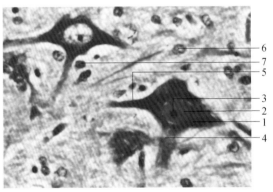

图 7-11　尼氏体（400×）
Fig. 7-11　Nissl body（400×）

⑫ 切片 12：轴 - 树突触（电镜）

材料与方法：小鼠大脑，电镜。

电镜观察：图 7-12 显示神经元的轴突终末（A）与树突（B）相接触，形成轴树突触。轴突终末内可见突触小泡（1），同时可见线粒体（2）。突触有突触前膜（3）、突触间隙（4）和突触后膜（5）组成。此突触前膜比后膜厚，为不对称突触。

12. Section 12: Axo-dendritic synapse (EM)

Materials and methods: Cereberum of the mouse, EM.

EM: Figure 7-12 shows an axo-dendritic synapse consists of an axon terminal (A) and dendrite (B). There are synaptic vesicles (1) in the axon terminal. A mitochondria (2) also can be found in this axon terminal. The synapse consists of a pre-synaptic membrane (3), a synaptic cleft (4), and a post-synaptic membrane (5). This presynaptic membrane is thicker than the posterior membrane, and therefore is an asymmetric synapse.

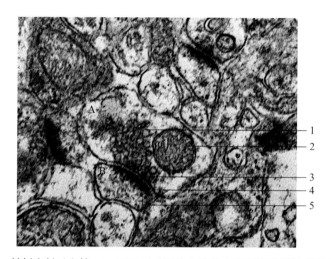

图 7-12　轴树突触（电镜，70 000×）（图片由清华大学医学院贾怡昌教授提供）
Fig. 7-12　axo-dendritic synapse (EM, 70 000×)(The photo is provided by Prof. Jia Yichang from School of Medicine, Tsinghua University)

【作业】

1. 绘图描述光镜下脊髓前角运动神经元的结构。
2. 绘图描述电镜下化学性突触的结构。

【Assignment】

1. Please draw the structure of the motor neurons in the anterior horn of the spinal cord under the LM.
2. Please draw the structure of chemical synapse under EM.

【思考题】

1. 试述一个多极神经元的形态结构。
2. 试述神经胶质细胞的分类。
3. 试述神经末梢的分类。
4. 说明化学突触的超微结构特点及信息传递过程。

【Questions】

1. To describe the morphological structure of a multipolar neuron.
2. To describe the types of neuroglial cells.

3. To describe the type of nerve ending.

4. To describe the ultrastructure of a chemical synapse and its process for information transfer.

【临床与科研联系英文阅读材料】
【English Reading Material for Correlations with Clinic and Scientific Research】

Amyotrophic lateral sclerosis (ALS) is a specific disorder that involves the death of neurons that control voluntary muscles. In some countries, the term motor neuron disease (MND) is commonly used, while others use that term for a group of five conditions of which ALS is the most common. ALS is characterized by stiff muscles, muscle twitching, and gradually worsening weakness due to muscles decreasing in size. This results in difficulty in speaking, swallowing, and eventually breathing.

（王大亮）

第8章 神经系统

Chapter 8 Nervous System

【实习内容】Contents of Observation

切片 Sections

观察切片	Observation Sections
1. 脊髓横切	1. Transversal section of spinal cord
2. 小脑	2. Cerebellum
3. 大脑	3. Cerebrum
4. 脊神经节	4. Spinal ganglia
5. 交感神经节	5. Sympathetic ganglia
示教切片	**Teaching Sections**
6. 脊髓（银染）	6. Spinal cord（silver staining）
7. 肌间神经丛	7. Myenteric plexus

【目的要求】

1. 掌握脊髓的构造。
2. 掌握小脑、大脑的结构分层特点。
3. 比较脊神经节、交感神经节的结构特点及区别，比较神经节节细胞与锥体细胞的结构不同。

【 Objective 】

1. To master the structure of spinal cord.

2. To master the layered structures of the cerebellum and cerebrum.

3. To compare the differences between spinal neuron ganglia and sympathetic ganglia. To compare the structural differences between ganglia cells and pyramid cells.

【 观察切片 】
【 Observation Sections 】

1 切片 1：脊髓

材料与方法：猫脊髓，HE 染色。

低倍镜观察：图 8-1a（20×）显示脊髓横断面，呈扁圆形，分为灰质和白质两个区域。灰质（实线）位于中央，呈 H 形，染色较暗。由较宽的前角（1）、较窄的后角（2）及灰质联合（3）三个部分组成，中央管（4）位于灰质联合内。白质位于周围，染色较淡，通常分为前索（5）、侧索（6）和后索（7）。贯穿脊髓的一条明显的、狭窄的裂缝为前正中裂（8）。后根（9）由感觉神经纤维组成，前根（10）主要由运动神经纤维组成。脊髓膜由内向外分为软脊膜（11），紧贴脊髓表面，富含血管；蛛网膜（12），可见脊髓的前根及后根的断面；硬脊膜（13），最外层的结缔组织膜（部分已脱落）。

1. Section 1: Spinal cord

Materials and methods: Spinal cord of the cat, HE staining.

LPM: Figure 8-1a (20×) shows the transvers section of spinal cord. It is oval shape, and is divided into two regions, gray matter and white matter. The gray matter is located in the center, with H-shape, darker staining. It consists of wider ventral horn (1), thinner dorsal horn (2), and grey commissure (3). The central canal (4) lies in the central commissure of gray matter. The peripheral white matter with a pale staining, generally consists of ventral funiculus (5), lateral funiculus (6),

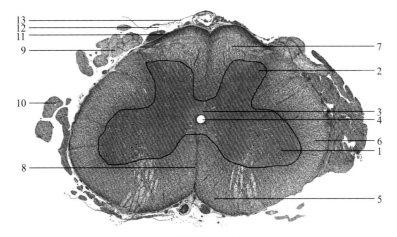

图 8-1a　脊髓横断面（20×）

Fig. 8-1a　Cross section of spinal cord (20×)

and dorsal funiculus (7). Throughout most the length of spinal cord, a narrow fissure is ventral median fissure (8). The dorsal root (9) consists of the sensory nerve fibers, but the ventral root (10) consists of the motor nerve fibers. Form inside to outside, the spinal cord is divided into pia mater (11), which is close to the surface of the spinal cord, with rich blood vessels; the arachnoid (12), visible at the anterior and posterior part of the spinal cord; the dura matter (13), the outermost layer of connective tissue membrane (part of it has fallen off).

高倍镜观察：在脊髓灰质前角部位（图 8-1b），可见许多散在神经细胞为前角运动神经元（1），体积较大。灰质区可见神经纤维网（2）包绕很多小神经元（3）和神经胶质细胞（4）。白质区（图 8-1c）主要由中央轴突、周围髓鞘溶解的有髓神经纤维（5）结构组成。从 α- 运动神经元发出的纵切有髓神经纤维（6）穿梭于白质。

HPM: In the ventral horn of gray matter of the spinal cord (Figure 8-1b), a lot of larger scattered ventral horn motor neurons (1) can be observed. There are a number of small neurons (2) and neuroglia cells (4) surrounding by the neuropil (3). The white matter (Figure 8-1c) prominently consists of central axons and myelinated nerve fibers (5), with dissolved peripheral myelin sheath. In addition, the medullated fibers (6) cut in longitudinal section extending from α-motor neuron passing through the whole white matter.

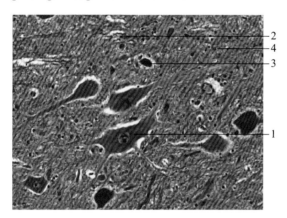
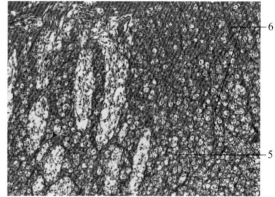

图 8-1b　脊髓灰质（400×）

Fig. 8-1b　Gray matter of the spinal cord (400×)

图 8-1c　脊髓白质（100×）

Fig. 8-1c　White matter of the spinal cord (100×)

❷ 切片 2：小脑

材料与方法：小鼠小脑，HE 染色。

低倍镜观察：图 8-2a 显示小脑的皮质由浅入深分为 3 层：分子层（1）、浦肯野细胞层（2）和颗粒层（3），（4）为小脑髓质。

高倍镜观察：图 8-2b 显示小脑分子层（1）显示为浅粉色，主要由大量无髓神经纤维和少量星形细胞、篮状细胞组成。颗粒层（2）细胞密集，由颗粒细胞和高尔基细胞组成，细胞核深染。分子层与颗粒层之间即为浦肯野细胞层（3），浦肯野细胞（4）为小脑最大的神经元。

2. Section 2: Cerebellum

Materials and methods: Cerebellum of the mouse, HE staining.

LPM: Figure 8-2a shows surface to deep, the cerebellar cortex from the shallower to the deep consisting of three layers: molecular layer (1), Purkinje cell layer (2), and granular layer (3), cerebellar medulla is shown (4).

HPM: Figure 8-2b shows the pale pink-stained molecular layer (1), which consists unmyelinated nerve fibers and a few stellate neurons, basket neurons. Granular cell layer (2) is dense, which consists of granular cells and Golgi cells with darker stained nuclei. Purkinje cell layer (3) is located between molecular layer and granular layer. The Purkinje cell (4) is the largest neuron of cerebellum.

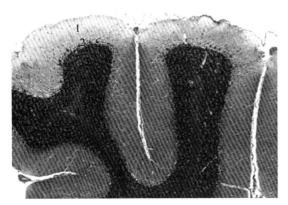

图 8-2a　小脑（100×）

Fig. 8-2a　Cerebellum (100×)

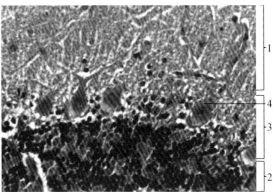

图 8-2b　小脑皮质（400×）

Fig. 8-2b　Cerebellar cortex (400×)

❸ 切片 3：大脑

材料与方法：小鼠大脑，HE 染色。

低倍镜观察：图 8-3a 显示大脑表面为软脑膜（↙），由薄层结缔组织组成，内含小血管。皮层由分子层（1）、外颗粒层（2）、外锥体细胞层（3）、内颗粒层（4）、内锥体细胞层（5）和多形细胞层（6）组成。（7）为大脑髓质。

3. Section 3: Cerebrum

Materials and methods: Cerebrum of the mouse, HE staining.

LPM: Figure 8-3a shows that the surface of cerebrum is pia mater (↙), which consists of thin layer of connective tissue, containing small blood vessel. The cerebrum cortex consists of molecular layer (1), external granular layer (2), external pyramidal layer (3), internal granular layer (4), internal pyramidal cell layer (5) and multiform cell layer (6). Cerebrum medulla is shown (7).

高倍镜观察：图 8-3b 显示大脑皮质局部。皮质内主要由各种类型神经细胞（1）和无髓神经纤维组成（2）。常规 HE 染色中各层细胞界限分界不清，图 8-3c 显示细胞间红色线样结构为无髓神经纤维（3）所在处，一些较大的锥体细胞（4）容易辨认。图 8-3d 显示大脑髓质，又称白质，主要由神经胶质细胞（5）和有髓神经纤维（6）组成。

HPM: Figure 8-3b shows the part of cerebrum cortex. The cortex consists prominently varieties of neurons (1), and unmyelinated nerve fibers (2). It is difficult to identify the boundary of each layer using general HE staining. In Figure 8-3c the red line-like structures in the intercellular matrix are unmyelinated nerve fibers (3). Some larger pyramidal neurons (4) can be easily observed. The Figure 8-3d shows the cerebrum medulla, which consists of neuroglia cells (5) and myelinated nerve fibers (6).

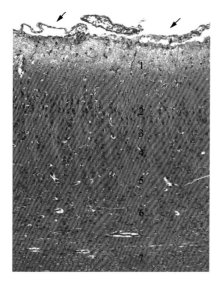

图 8-3a 大脑（20×）
Fig. 8-3a Cerebrum (20×)

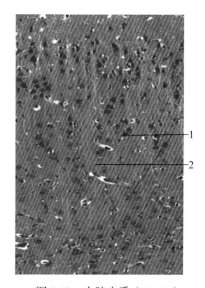

图 8-3b 大脑皮质（100×）
Fig. 8-3b Cerebrum cortex (100×)

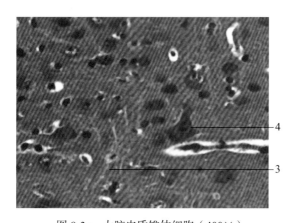

图 8-3c 大脑皮质锥体细胞（400×）
Fig. 8-3c Pyramidal cells in cerebrum cortex (400×)

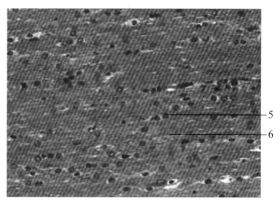

图 8-3d 大脑髓质（200×）
Fig. 8-3d Cerebrum medulla (200×)

❹ 切片 4：脑脊神经节

材料与方法：人脑脊神经节，HE 染色。

低倍镜观察：神经节是中枢神经系统以外的神经细胞聚集体。脊神经节的神经元多为假单极神经元。图 8-4a 显示脊神经节。其表面为致密结缔组织组成的被膜（1）。脊神经节含有不同大小的假单极神经元的胞体（2）。节细胞胞体通常排列成行或聚集成束。行间红染的神经纤维（3）由节细胞的突起所组成。

4. Section 4: Brain and spinal ganglia

Materials and methods: Brain and spinal ganglia of human, HE staining.

LPM: Ganglia are discrete aggregations of neuron cell bodies located outside the central nervous system. Spinal ganglion neurons are mostly pseudo-monopole neurons. Figure 8-4a shows the spinal ganglia. Its surface is covered by a connective tissue capsule (1). The spinal ganglia contain various sized perikarya (2) of pseudo-unipolar neurons. The perikarya are generally arranged in rows or clusters. The red-staining nerve fibers (3) between cell-rows consist of processes of ganglia cells.

高倍镜观察：图 8-4b 显示节细胞，部分节细胞胞体中可见较大的细胞核（1）及明显的核仁（2）。紧靠节细胞外面的一层扁平细胞为卫星细胞（3），也称被囊细胞。在卫星细胞外面，有结缔组织包绕（4）。神经纤维束（5）中可见有髓神经纤维的施万细胞核（6）。

HPM: Figure 8-4b shows the ganglion cells, some of which show big nucleus (1) and prominent nucleolus (2). The flat cells, which are surrounding the ganglion cell, are satellite cells (3), also called capsule cells. Outside of satellite cells is surrounded by connective tissue (4). Schwann cell nuclei (6) can be observed within the bundles of myelinated nerve fibers (5).

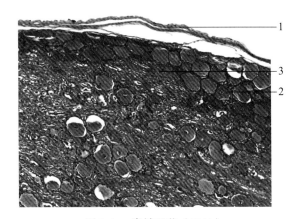 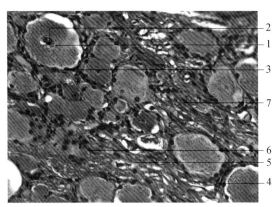

| 图 8-4a　脊神经节（40×） | 图 8-4b　脊神经节（400×） |
| Fig. 8-4a　Spinal ganglia (40×) | Fig. 8-4b　Spinal ganglia (400×) |

⑤ 切片 5：交感神经节

材料与方法：人交感神经节，HE 染色。

低倍镜观察：图 8-5a 显示交感神经节，其表面被覆结缔组织构成的被膜（1）。节内分布较大的交感神经节细胞（2），节细胞间可见成束排列的神经纤维（3）。

5. Section 5: Sympathetic ganglion

Materials and methods: Sympathetic ganglion of human, HE staining.

LPM: Figure 8-5a shows the sympathetic ganglion. Its surface is covered by connective tissue (1). Ganglion contains a number of larger ganglion cells (2). The nerve fibers (3) are arranged in bundle between ganglion cells.

高倍镜观察：图 8-5b 显示交感神经节细胞为多极神经元（1），细胞胞体呈圆形或多边形。胞质内可见嗜碱性的尼氏体（2），较大的核（3）及明显的核仁（4）。节细胞周围有卫星细胞和结缔组织所包绕，但数量较少。卫星细胞的核（5）呈圆形，而结缔组织细胞核（6）呈梭形。神经节内可见到有髓神经纤维（7）存在。

HPM: Figure 8-5b shows that the sympathetic ganglion cell is multipolar neuron (1), with a round or polygonal perikaryon. In perikaryon, there is basophilic Nissl body (2), a large nucleus (3) and prominent nucleolus (4). The perikaryon is surrounded by a few satellite cells and connective tissue. The nucleus of satellite cell (5) is round-shape, but the nucleus of connective tissue (6) is fusiform. The myelinated nerve fibers (7) are present in the ganglion.

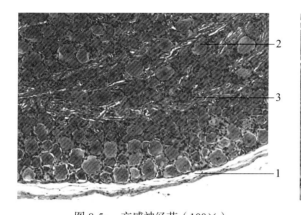

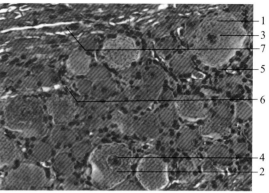

图 8-5a　交感神经节（100×）

Fig. 8-5a　Sympathetic ganglion (100×)

图 8-5b　节细胞（400×）

Fig. 8-5b　Ganglion cells (400×)

【示教切片】
【Teaching Sections】

6 切片 6：脊髓横切（银染）

材料与方法：猫脊髓，银染。

低倍镜观察：图 8-6a 显示横断面下脊髓表面完整的硬脊膜（1）、蛛网膜下腔（2）及软脊膜（3）的结构。

6. Section 6: Cross section of spinal cord (silver staining)

Materials and methods: Spinal Cord of the cat, paraffin embedding, silver staining.

LPM: Figure 8-6a shows the intact dura matter (1), subarachnoid space (2), and pie matter (3) on the surface of spinal cord in cross section.

低倍镜观察：图 8-6b 显示银染条件下，神经元（1）显示为棕黄色，神经纤维的轴突（2）显示为棕黑色，有髓神经纤维的髓鞘（3）溶解呈透明区域。从前角的 α- 运动神经元发

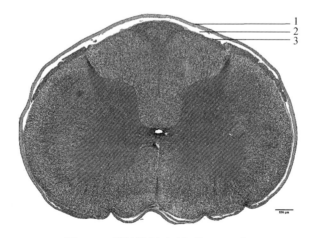

图 8-6a　脊髓横断面（银染，20×）

Fig. 8-6a　Cross section of spinal cord (Silver Staining, 20×)

出的纵切的有髓神经纤维（4）贯穿白质，形成前根（5）。脊神经的后根由脊神经节内感觉神经元的轴突组成。

LPM: Figure 8-6b shows that using the silver staining, the neuron (1) is showed as pale brown, the axons (2) of nerve fibers as black, and the sheath (3) of myelinated nerve fiber as clear due to the sheath dissolution. The longitudinal myelinated nerve fibers (4) extending from α-motor neurons of ventral horn run through the white matter and form the ventral root (5). The dorsal root of spinal cord consists of the axons of sensory neurons within spinal ganglion.

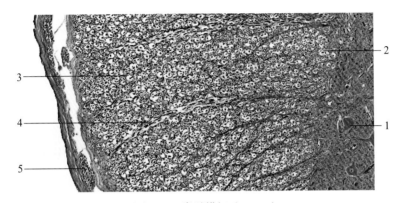

图 8-6b　脊髓横切（100×）

Fig. 8-6b　Cross section of spinal cord (100×)

🄻 切片 7：肌间神经丛

材料与方法：人小肠，HE 染色。

高倍镜观察：图 8-7 显示肠道环行肌（A）和纵行肌层（B）之间存在神经丛（1），神经丛（奥尔巴克神经丛）主要由神经细胞（2）和一些神经胶质细胞（3）组成。

7. Section 7: Myenteric nerve plexus

Materials and methods: Human intestine, HE staining.

HPM: Figure 8-7 shows the myenteric nerve plexus (1) between the circular (A) and

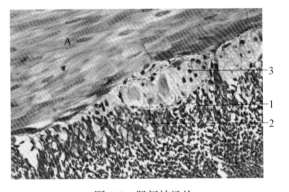

图 8-7　肌间神经丛

Fig. 8-7　Myenteric nerve plexus

longitudinal (B) muscles layers of the intestine. The plexus (Auerbath plexus) mainly consists of neurons (2) and glia cells (3).

【作业】

绘图描述大脑皮质结构。

【Assignment】

Please draw the cortical structure of the cerebrum.

【思考题】

1. 描述脊髓的组成及结构特点。
2. 小脑皮质可分为几层？各层主要由哪些神经元组成？
3. 大脑皮质可分为几层？各层主要由哪些神经元组成？
4. 血 - 脑脊液屏障包括哪些结构？

【Questions】

1. Please describe the composition and structures of spinal cord.
2. How many layers has the cerebellum cortex? what are the main neurons at each layer?
3. How many layers has the cerebrum cortex? what are the main neurons at each layer?
4. What is the composition of blood-brain barrier (BBB) ?

【临床与科研联系英文阅读材料】
【English Reading Material for Correlations with Clinic and Scientific Research】

Parkinson's disease, a crippling disease related to the absence of dopamine in certain regions of the brain, is characterized by muscular rigidity, constant tremor, bradykinesia (slow movement), and finally, a mask-like face and difficult voluntary movement. Because dopamine cannot cross the blood-brain barrier, therapy is administered as L-dopa (levodopa), which relieves the motor abnormalities temporarily, although the neurons in the affected area continue to die. Effort to transplant fetal adrenal gland tissue into persons with this disease have provided only transient relief. The therapeutic grafting of genetically modified cells capable of secreting dopamine will perhaps allow the establishment of synaptic connections to cells in the corpus striatum of the brain where dopamine is needed.

（王大亮）

第 9 章 循环系统

Chapter 9 Circulatory System

【实习内容】Contents of Observation

切片 Sections

观察切片	Observation Sections
1. 股动脉和股静脉	1. Femoral artery and vein
2. 大动脉	2. Aorta
3. 心室壁	3. Ventricle
4. 小动脉和小静脉	4. Small artery and small vein
示教切片	**Teaching Sections**
5. 连续性毛细血管（电镜）	5. Continuous capillary（EM）

【目的要求】

1. 掌握心脏壁的结构特点，在光镜下正确辨认。
2. 掌握大动脉、中动脉和中静脉的结构特点，在光镜下正确区分。
3. 熟悉毛细血管的光镜和电镜结构。

【Objective】

1. To master structural characteristics of the heart wall and correctly identify them under light microscopy.

2. To master morphological features of large artery, medium-sized artery and medium-sized vein, and correctly distinguish them under light microscopy.

3. To be familiar with structural features of capillary under light microscopy or electron microscopy.

【观察切片】
【Observation Sections】

① 切片1：中动脉和中静脉

材料与方法：动物股动脉和股静脉，HE 染色。

低倍镜观察：图 9-1a 显示中动脉内膜（1）、中膜（2）、外膜（3）。在内膜与中膜交界处有一条波浪状、亮粉红色的内弹性膜（4）。外膜与中膜相连处有外弹性膜（5），外弹性膜不如内弹性膜明显。图 9-1b 显示中静脉内膜（1）、中膜（2）、外膜（3）。中静脉的三层膜均较动脉的薄。

1. Section 1: Medium-sized artery and medium-sized vein

Materials and methods: Animal femoral artery and vein, HE staining.

LPM: Figure 9-1a shows that the wall of medium-sized artery divided into three layers: tunica intima (1), tunica media (2) and tunica adventitia (3). The internal elastic lamina (4) is prominent; appears as a wavy, bright pink, junction between the tunica intima and the tunica media. An external elastic lamina (5) is situated between the tunica media and the tunica adventitia. Figure 9-1b shows the medium-sized vein. The wall of the medium-sized vein consists of three layers, tunica intima (1), tunica media (2) and tunica adventitia (3). The three layers of medium-sized vein are all thinner than those of medium-sized artery.

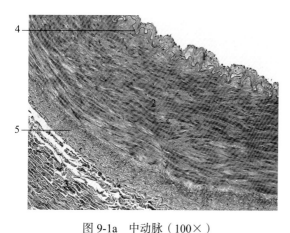

图 9-1a　中动脉（100×）
Fig. 9-1a　Medium-sized artery (100×)

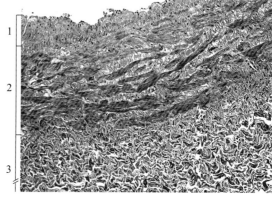

图 9-1b　中静脉（100×）
Fig. 9-1b　Medium-sized vein (100×)

高倍镜观察：图 9-1c 显示中动脉内膜分为三层：内皮（1）、内皮下层（2）、内弹性膜（3）。中膜（4）由多层较密集排列的环形平滑肌组成，平滑肌纤维之间有弹性纤维和胶原纤维。图 9-1d 显示中静脉内膜（1）和中膜（2）。内弹性膜不明显。

HPM: Figure 9-1c shows that the tunica intima of medium-sized artery, which consists of three layers, endothelium (1), subendothelial layer (2) and internal elastic lamina (3). The tunica media (4) is comprised of many layers of more densely arrayed and circumferential smooth muscle cells. Among muscle cells, small amounts of elastic fibers and collagen fibers are observed. Figure 9-1d shows that tunica intima (1), tunica media (2) of the medium-sized vein. The internal elastic membrane is not clear.

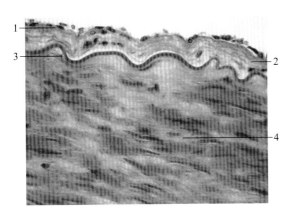

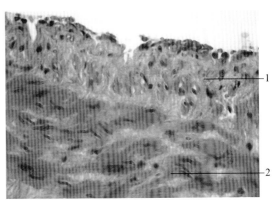

图 9-1c 中动脉（400×）

Fig. 9-1c Medium-sized artery (400×)

图 9-1d 中静脉（400×）

Fig. 9-1d Medium-sized vein (400×)

❷ 切片 2：大动脉

材料与方法：人主动脉壁，HE 染色。

低倍镜观察：图 9-2a 显示管壁分为三层：内膜（1）、中膜（2）、外膜（3），三层膜分界不明显。图 9-2b 显示内膜（1）和中膜（2），中膜可见多层亮红色折光性强的弹性膜（3），呈波浪状。

2. Section 2: Large artery

Materials and methods: Human aorta, HE staining.

LPM: Figure 9-2a shows that the wall of the aorta is divided into three layers, tunica intima (1), tunica media (2) and tunica adventitia (3). The borders of three tunics of the wall are not distinctive. Figure 9-2b shows tunica intima (1) and tunica media (2). The elastic lamina (3), with many wavy, bright red and refractile lines, are seen in the tunica media.

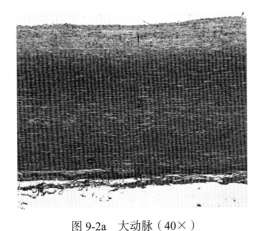

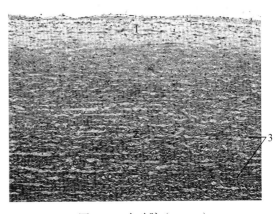

图 9-2a 大动脉（40×）

Fig. 9-2a Large artery (40×)

图 9-2b 大动脉（100×）

Fig. 9-2b Large artery (100×)

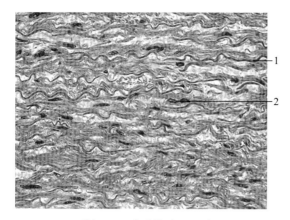

图 9-2c　大动脉（400×）

Fig. 9-2c　Large artery (400×)

高倍镜观察：图 9-2c 显示大动脉中膜含有多层波浪状弹性膜（1），其间夹有平滑肌纤维（2）和较细的弹性纤维。

HPM: Figure 9-2c shows that the tunica media contains numerous wavy-like elastic laminae (1), alternating with smooth muscle cells (2) and elastic fibers.

❸ 切片 3：心脏

材料与方法：动物心壁，HE 染色。

低倍镜观察：图 9-3a 显示心内膜（1）和部分心肌膜（2）。心内膜较薄，腔面为内皮（3）。心肌膜较厚，主要由心肌纤维（4）组成。心肌纤维呈螺旋状排列，故在切片中可见肌纤维的纵切、横切及斜切面。图 9-3b 显示心肌膜（1）和心外膜（2），心外膜染色较浅，主要为结缔组织，可见小血管（3）和脂肪细胞（4）。

3. Section 3: Heart

Materials and methods: Animal heart wall (ventricle), HE staining.

LPM: Figure 9-3a shows endocardium (1) and myocardium (2). The endocardium is thin, and which the innermost layer is endothelium (3). The myocardium is thick and consists mainly of cardiac muscle fibers (4) arranged in a complex helical pattern. Therefore, the longitudinal, cross and oblique sections may be seen in the specimen. Figure 9-3b shows myocardium (1) and epicardium (2). The epicardium is stained pale and consists of connective tissue that contains small blood vessels (3) and adipocytes (4).

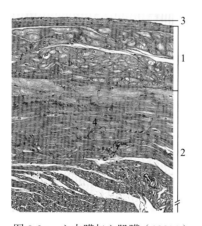

图 9-3a　心内膜与心肌膜（100×）

Fig. 9-3a　Endocardium and myocardium (100×)

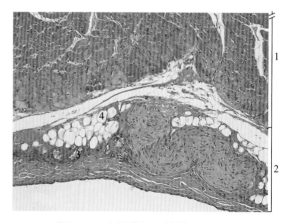

图 9-3b　心肌膜与心外膜（100×）

Fig. 9-3b　Myocardium and epicardium (100×)

高倍镜观察：图 9-3c 显示心内膜与部分心肌膜。腔面为内皮（1），内皮下为较细密的结缔组织，即内皮下层（2），其深面为心内膜下层。心内膜下层内可见浦肯野纤维（束细胞）（3），比一般心肌纤维（4）粗短，肌浆丰富，肌丝少且位于细胞的周边，故细胞中央染色较浅；核大，1～2 个，居中。图 9-3d 显示心内膜（1）与部分心肌膜（2）。心肌膜主要由心肌纤维（3）组成，其间有少量结缔组织和丰富的毛细血管。心肌纤维纵切面为短圆柱状，有分支和不明显的横纹；核卵圆，位于肌纤维中央；相邻心肌纤维连接处可见深红色闰盘（4）。

HPM: Figure 9-3c shows endocardium and partial myocardium. The endothelium (1) is seen lining the ventricle lumen. Beneath the endothelium is the subendothelial layer (2) of connective tissue. The underlying subendocardial layer contains Purkinje fibers (3). Purkinje fiber is shorter than typical cardiac muscle cell (4). It is rich in sarcoplasm, with only a few myofibrils located peripherally. So that, the center part of Purkinje fiber is stained pale. One or two spherical nuclei are located in the cell center. Figure 9-3d shows endocardium (1) and partial myocardium (2). The myocardium is mainly composed of cardiac muscle fibers (3). There is a small amount of connective tissue and rich capillaries between muscle fibers. In longitudinal section, cardiac muscle fiber appears as short cylinder with branches. Indistinct transverse striations are seen in the muscle fiber. Ovoid nucleus is located in the center of the muscle fiber. The dark red intercalated disks (4) between the neighboring muscle fibers are observed.

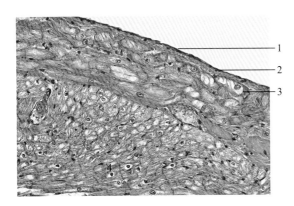

图 9-3c　心内膜与心肌膜（400×）

Fig. 9-3c　Endocardium and myocardium (400×)

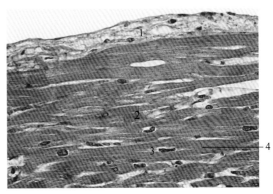

图 9-3d　心内膜与心肌膜（400×）

Fig. 9-3d　Endocardium and myocardium (400×)

❹ 切片 4：小动脉和小静脉

材料与方法：动物心壁，HE 染色。

低倍镜观察：图 9-4，可见在结缔组织内，壁厚、腔小而规则的为小动脉（1）；壁薄、腔大而不规则者为小静脉（2）。小动脉管壁的三层结构比较完整，内膜的内皮下可见明显的内弹性膜，中膜为 4～5 层环行平滑肌，外膜为结缔组织，外膜与周围结缔组织无明显分界。小静脉的内皮细胞核为扁椭圆形，内皮外可见 1～2 层排列稀疏的平滑肌细胞。

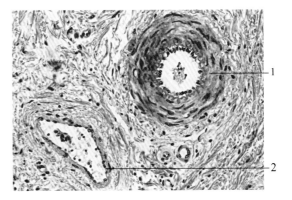

图 9-4　小动脉和小静脉（200×）

Fig. 9-4　Small artery and small vein (200×)

4. Section 4: Small artery and small vein

Materials and methods: Animal heart wall (ventricle), HE staining.

LPM: Figure 9-4, in the connective tissue, the vessel with thick wall, small and regular lumen is the small artery (1). The vessel with thin wall, large and irregular lumen is the small vein (2). The wall of the small artery can be divided into three distinctive layers. In tunica intima, the internal elastic lamina is prominent. The tunica media is composed of 4-5 layers of circular arranged smooth muscle cells. The tunica adventitia consists of connective tissue. The tunica adventitia is continuous with the surrounding connective tissue. In the small vein, the nuclei of endothelial cells are oval. Beneath the endothelium are 1-2 layers of loosely-arranged smooth muscle cells. There is no distinct boundary between the adventitia and the peripheral connective tissue.

【示教切片】
【Teaching Sections】

⑤ 切片 5: 连续毛细血管（电镜）

电镜下，毛细血管可分为 3 型，分别为连续毛细血管、有孔毛细血管和血窦。1）图 9-5 显示连续毛细血管，可见内皮细胞间有紧密连接（1），内皮外的基膜（2）完整，胞质中有许多吞饮小泡（3），（4）为毛细血管内皮细胞核。2）有孔毛细血管：内皮细胞不含核的部分很薄，有许多贯穿细胞的窗孔，孔上有隔膜封闭。内皮细胞间也有紧密连接，基膜完整。3）血窦也称窦状毛细血管：管腔大而不规则，内皮细胞之间常有较大的间隙，基膜不完整或无。

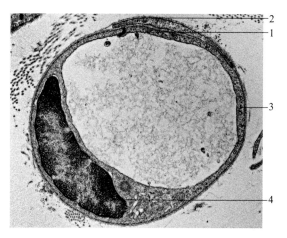

图 9-5 连续毛细血管（25000×）
Fig. 9-5 Continuous capillary (25000×)

5. Section 5: Continuous capillaries (EM)

Under EM, capillaries are classified into three types: continuous capillaries, fenestrated capillaries and sinusoidal capillaries. 1) Figure 9-5 shows the continuous capillaries. There are tight junction (1) between endothelial cells, complete basement membrane (2) outside the endothelium, many pinocytotic vesicles in the cytoplasm (3), and capillary endothelial nuclei (4). 2) Fenestrated capillaries, in which the endothelial cells are perforated by fenestrae. The fenestrae may be open or covered by thin diaphragms. The cells attach tightly with each other by tight junctions. The basal lamina is continuous. 3) Sinusoidal capillaries, also called sinusoids. This capillary has wide and irregular lumen and follows a tortuous path. There are gaps between the endothelial cells. The basal lamina is often discontinuous or absence.

【作业】

绘图描述中动脉的高倍镜结构。

【Assignment】

Drawing to describe morphological structures of the medium-sized artery under high power microscopy.

【思考题】

1．在光镜下如何区别中动脉与中静脉?
2．大动脉为何又称弹性动脉? 其结构与中动脉有何异同?
3．心脏壁的结构有何特点? 浦肯野纤维与一般心肌纤维有何异同?

【Questions】

1. How to distinguish medium-sized artery from medium-sized vein under light microscopy?

2. Large arteries are also called elastic arteries, Why? What are the similarities and differences comparing large arteries with medium-sized arteries?

3. What are the structural features of the heart wall? What are the similarities and differences comparing Purkinje fibers with typical cardiac muscle fibers?

【临床与科研联系英文阅读材料】
【English Reading Material for Correlations with Clinic and Scientific Research】

Tumor growth, metastasis and recurrence are closely related to the new blood vessel formation. The formation of new blood vessels not only provides ongoing nutrition and oxygen for tumor growth and takes away metabolites at the same time, but also transports tumor cells to target organs, which provides a necessary condition for tumor metastasis. Traditional point of view considers that tumor blood supply patterns mainly include vasculogenesis and angiogenesis, and their common characteristic is endothelial cell-dependent. Prior anti-vascular therapy just focused on vascular endothelial cells. The vasculogenic mimicry (VM) was not taken into consideration, which resulted in poor therapeutic effects. VM is the ability of aggressive cancer cells to acquire an altered phenotype and to form a tumor cell-lined vasculature. As a brand new pattern of the tumor blood supply, VM does not depend on the endothelial cells. Tumor cells have direct access to the bloodstream through the tumor cell-lined vessels and tend to spread aggressively due to VM formation. VM is usually observed in high-grade invasive tumors and is associated with poor prognosis. VM might also be partly responsible for resistance to antiangiogenic drugs.

（郭晓霞　尚宏伟）

第10章 免疫系统

Chapter 10 Immune System

【实习内容】Contents of Observation

切片 Sections

观察切片	Observation Sections
1. 胸腺	1. Thymus
2. 淋巴结	2. Lymph node
3. 脾	3. Spleen
4. 腭扁桃体	4. Palatine tonsil

【目的要求】

1. 掌握胸腺的结构特点并正确辨认。
2. 掌握淋巴结的结构特点并正确辨认。
3. 掌握脾的结构特点并正确辨认。
4. 了解腭扁桃体的组织结构。

【Objective】

1. To master structural characteristics of thymus, and correctly identify it under light microscope.

2. To master morphological features of lymph nodes, and correctly identify them under light microscope.

3. To master morphological features of spleen, and correctly identify it under light microscope.

4. To understand structural features of palatine tonsils.

【观察切片】
【Observation Sections】

1 切片 1：胸腺

材料与方法：胎儿胸腺，HE 染色。

低倍镜观察：图 10-1a 显示被膜（1）和小叶间隔（2）为粉红色薄层结缔组织，小叶间隔将实质分成许多不完全分隔的胸腺小叶。皮质（3）位于小叶周边，细胞密集，呈强嗜碱性染色。髓质（4）位于小叶深部，细胞较少，染色较浅。相邻小叶的髓质相互连接，其中可见染成红色的胸腺小体（5）。

1. Section 1: Thymus

Materials and methods: Fetus thymus, HE staining.

LPM: Figure 10-1a shows that the capsule (1) is composed of a thin layer of connective tissue which is pink-staining. Interbobular septum penetrates into the thymus parenchyma and form interlobular septum (2), dividing the parenchyma into incomplete thymic lobules. The cortex (3) is located in the periphery of the lobule. It contains highly concentrated thymocytes, and is intensely basophilic. The medulla (4) is located in the center of the lobule. It is less cellular and pale-staining. The medulla of adjacent lobules is in continuity. The red-staining thymic corpuscles (Hassall's corpuscles) (5) can be seen in the medulla.

图 10-1b 显示皮质（1）由密集的胸腺细胞和少量的胸腺上皮细胞组成。胸腺细胞体积小，胞质嗜碱性，核染色深。胸腺上皮细胞核大而染色浅，核仁明显。髓质（2）胸腺上皮细胞较多，淋巴细胞较少，可见散在的胸腺小体（3）。胸腺小体大小不等，由数层扁平的胸腺上皮细胞呈同心圆排列而成；小体外周的细胞较幼稚，胞质嗜酸性，核明显；中央的细胞呈均质状、嗜酸性，核消失。

Figure 10-1b shows that the cortex (1) is comprised of many thymocytes and fewer thymic epithelial cells. Thymocytes are small and basophilic, their nuclei are dark-staining. The nuclei of thymic epithelial cells are large and pale-staining, with prominent nucleoli. The medulla (2) contains

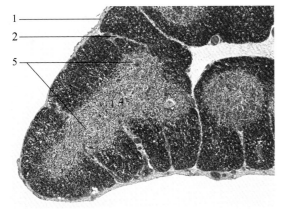

图 10-1a　胸腺（40×）

Fig. 10-1a　Thymus（40×）

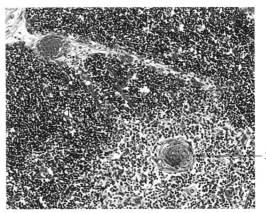

图 10-1b　胸腺（100×）

Fig. 10-1b　Thymus（100×）

many thymic epithelial cells and fewer lymphocytes. There are thymic corpuscles (3) in the medulla. The thymic corpuscles are spherical bodies of different sizes, which are composed of concentrically arranged thymic epithelial cells. The central cells often degenerate, the cytoplasm is eosinophilic, and the nucleus is not seen.

❷ 切片 2：淋巴结

材料与方法：人或动物淋巴结，HE 染色。

低倍镜观察：图 10-2a 显示被膜（1）由薄层致密结缔组织构成，有的部位可见输入淋巴管（2）。皮质位于被膜下方，由浅层皮质、副皮质区（3）和皮质淋巴窦（4）构成。浅层皮质由弥散淋巴组织和淋巴小结组成。弥散淋巴组织分布于被膜下淋巴窦周围和淋巴小结之间。淋巴小结是淋巴组织密集形成的球形结构，有的淋巴小结中央色浅，为生发中心（5），周围有色深的小结帽（6）。副皮质区是位于皮质深层的弥散淋巴组织。皮质淋巴窦是位于被膜下和小梁周围的间隙，染色较浅。图 10-2b 显示淋巴结髓质，位于淋巴结中央，由髓索（1）和髓窦（2）构成。髓索是不规则的条索状淋巴组织，染色较深，相互联结成网，网间间隙为髓窦，染色浅，腔大而不规则。可见结缔组织形成的小梁（3）。

2. Section 2: Lymph node

Materials and methods: Lymph node of human or animal, HE staining.

LPM: Figure 10-2a shows that the capsule (1) is composed of dense connective tissue. The sections of afferent lymphatic vessels (2) can be found in the capsule. The cortex is located beneath the capsule and includes superficial cortex, paracortex zone (3) and cortical sinus (4). The superficial cortex consists of diffuse lymphoid tissue and lymphoid nodules. The diffuse lymphoid tissue is distributed around the subcapsular sinus and among lymphoid nodules. The lymphoid nodule is spherical, dense lymphoid tissue. The central region in some nodules is stained pale, called the germinal center (5). The top of the nodule has a dark-staining cap (6). The paracortex zone is diffuse lymphoid tissue lying in the deep portion of the cortex. The cortical sinuses are pale-staining and distributed beneath the capsule or at the periphery of the trabeculae. Figure 10-2b shows that the medulla is located in the central part of the lymph node and consists of medullary cords (1) and medullary sinuses (2). The medullary cords are dark-staining, irregular cords formed by lymphoid tissue. They connect with

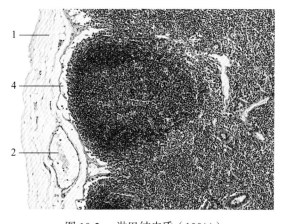
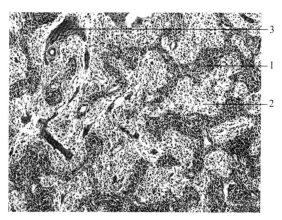

图 10-2a 淋巴结皮质（100×）
Fig. 10-2a Cortex of lymph node (100×)

图 10-2b 淋巴结髓质（100×）
Fig. 10-2b Medulla of lymph node (100×)

each other to form a network. The medullary sinuses are light-staining structures located among the medullary cords. Their lumens are big and irregular. The trabeculae can be seen (3).

高倍镜观察：图 10-2c 显示淋巴结副皮质区（1），可见高内皮微静脉（2），内皮细胞呈立方或柱状，可见正在穿越内皮的淋巴细胞。图 10-2d 显示淋巴结髓质，髓索（1）主要含浆细胞、B 细胞和巨噬细胞。髓窦（2）窦壁由扁平的内皮细胞（3）围成，窦腔中可见浅染的网状细胞（4），其间有淋巴细胞和体积较大且胞质嗜酸性的巨噬细胞。

HPM: Figure 10-2c shows the paracortex zone (1) of lymph node. The high endothelial venules (2) are observed, where the endothelial cells are cuboidal or columnar. Lymphocytes passing through the wall of the venule may be seen. Figure 10-2d shows the medulla of lymph node. The medullary cords (1) consist mainly of plasma cells, B lymphocytes and macrophages. The wall of the medullary sinus (2) is lined by flattened endothelial cells (3). The light-staining reticular cells (4), lymphocytes and macrophages can be found in the lumen of the sinus.

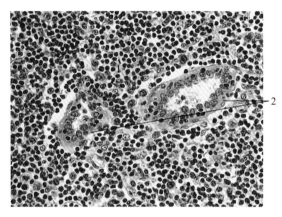

图 10-2c   淋巴结副皮质区（400×）

Fig. 10-2c   Paracortex zone of lymph node (400×)

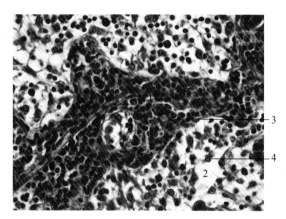

图 10-2d   淋巴结髓质（400×）

Fig. 10-2d   Medulla of lymph node (400×)

❸ 切片 3：脾

材料与方法：人或动物脾，HE 染色。

低倍镜观察：图 10-3a 显示脾被膜（1）较厚，由致密结缔组织构成，表面覆以间皮，内含平滑肌。被膜伸入实质形成小梁（2），有的内含血管。白髓（3）呈紫蓝色，由动脉周围淋巴鞘、脾小结、边缘区组成。红髓（4）由脾索和脾血窦组成。图 10-3b 显示脾白髓，中央动脉（1）周围较密集的淋巴组织为动脉周围淋巴鞘（2），脾小结（3）位于其一侧，两者之间没有明显的界线，由于切面不同，可呈圆形、椭圆形或不规则形。有的小结中央可见生发中心（4）。位于白髓和红髓交界处的狭窄区域是边缘区（5），此区淋巴细胞分布较稀疏。

3. Section 3: Spleen

Materials and methods: Spleen of human or animal, HE staining.

LPM: Figure 10-3a shows that the capsule (1) of the spleen is thick. It is composed of dense connective tissue, smooth muscle, and covered by mesothelium. The connective tissue extends into the spleen parenchyma to form trabeculae (2). Small arteries and veins can be found in the trabeculae. The white pulp (3) is blue-staining. It is composed of periarterial lymphatic sheath, splenic corpuscle and marginal zone. The red pulp (4) is made of splenic cords and splenic sinuses. Figure 10-3b shows the white pulp, around a central artery (1) is a cuff of lymphocytes, a periarterial lymphatic sheath (2). The splenic corpuscle (3) is round or oval in shape, located beside the periarterial lymphatic sheath. The germinal center (4) can be seen in some nodules. The marginal zone (5) lies the narrow area between the white pulp and the red pulp, consisting of loosely-arranged lymphocytes.

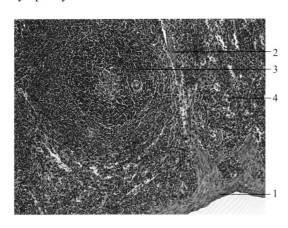

图 10-3a　脾（100×）

Fig. 10-3a　Spleen (100×)

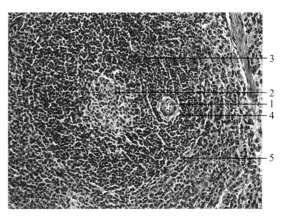

图 10-3b　脾白髓（200×）

Fig. 10-3b　White pulp of spleen (200×)

高倍镜观察：图 10-3c 显示红髓（1）和部分白髓（2）。红髓分布于白髓之间，以及白髓与小梁之间，呈红色，由脾索和脾血窦构成。脾索（3）位于脾血窦之间，由淋巴组织构成，呈不规则条索状，内含许多血细胞。脾血窦（4）腔较大而不规则，有的含大量血细胞，有的空虚。血窦壁衬杆状的内皮细胞，核圆形，凸向窦腔。

HPM: Figure 10-3c shows red pulp (1) and part of white pulp (2). The red pulp stains red. It is composed of splenic cords and splenic sinuses. The splenic cords (3) are composed of irregular lymphoid tissue strands with various types of blood cells. The splenic sinuses (4) are sinusoid with big irregular lumen, which occupy the spaces between the splenic cords. The wall of the sinus is composed of rod-shaped endothelial cells with round nuclei, which protrude into sinus cavity.

❹ 切片 4：腭扁桃体

材料与方法：人腭扁桃体，HE 染色。

低倍镜观察：图 10-4，扁桃体表面被覆未角化的复层扁平上皮（1），上皮向深部凹陷形成许多隐窝（2）。上皮下及隐窝周围的固有层内有大量淋巴小结（3）和弥散淋巴组织（4）。淋巴组织深面粉红色的结缔组织为被膜，被膜下方可见黏液腺。

4. Section 4: Palatine tonsil

Materials and methods: Human palatine tonsil, HE staining.

LPM: Figure 10-4, the palatine tonsil is covered by nonkeratinized stratified squamous epithelium (1). The epithelium invaginates to form many crypts (2). The lamina propria beneath the epithelium and surrounding the crypts contains many lymphoid nodules (3) and diffuse lymphoid tissue (4). Under the lymphoid tissue, the pink-staining connective tissue membrane can be found,

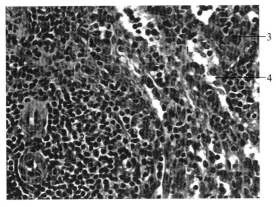

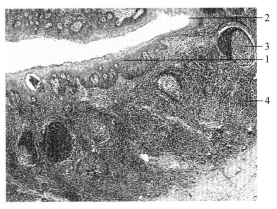

图 10-3c　脾红髓（400×）
Fig. 10-3c　Red pulp of spleen (400×)

图 10-4　腭扁桃体（40×）
Fig. 10-4　Palatine tonsil (40×)

under which are some mucous glands.

【作业】

绘图描述淋巴结的低倍镜或高倍镜结构。

【Assignment】

Draw to describe the morphological structures of lymph node under low or high power microscope.

【思考题】

1．T 细胞分化发育成熟的场所在哪里？主要分布在周围淋巴器官的哪些区域？
2．简述淋巴小结和弥散淋巴组织的结构特点。
3．淋巴结与脾的结构和功能有何异同？

【Questions】

1. In which organ do T-cells differentiate and mature? In peripheral lymphatic organs, where are T-cells mostly located?

2. Describe the structural features of lymphoid nodule and diffuse lymphoid tissue.

3. What are the similarities and differences in structures and functions between lymph node and spleen?

【临床与科研联系英文阅读材料】
【English Reading Material for Correlations with Clinic and Scientific Research】

Regulatory T (Treg) cells express Foxp3 transcription factor and control homeostasis of the immune system, antigenic responses to commensal and pathogenic microbiota, and immune responses to self and tumor antigens. The Treg cells differentiate in the thymus, along with conventional CD4$^+$ T cells, in the processes of positive and negative selections. Another class of Treg cells is generated in peripheral tissues by inducing Foxp3 expression in conventional CD4$^+$ T cells in response to antigenic stimulation. Both thymic and peripheral generation of Treg cells depend on the recognition of peptide/MHC ligands by the T-cell receptors (TCR), which is expressed on thymic Treg precursors or peripheral conventional CD4$^+$ T cells.

（郭晓霞　尚宏伟）

第 11 章 皮 肤

Chapter ⑪ Skin

【实习内容】Contents of Observation

切片　Sections

观察切片	Observe Sections
1. 指皮	1. Skin of finger
2. 背皮	2. Dorsal skin
3. 头皮	3. Scalp

【目的要求】

1. 掌握皮肤的组成和结构。
2. 掌握汗腺和毛囊的结构。
3. 了解指皮和体皮（背皮）的区别。
4. 了解毛发、立毛肌以及皮脂腺的结构。

【Objective】

1. To master the constituent and structure characteristics of skin.
2. To master the structure characteristics of sweat gland and hair follicle.
3. To understand the differences between the skin of finger and the skin of body.
4. To understand the structure of hair, arrector pili muscle and sebaceous gland.

【观察切片】
【Observation Sections】

❶ 切片1：手指皮肤

材料与方法：人手指皮肤，HE 染色。

低倍镜观察：图 11-1a 显示手指皮肤，由表皮（1）和真皮（2）构成，表皮为角化的复层鳞状上皮。真皮为致密结缔组织，可分为紧贴表皮的乳头层和其下方的网织层，两者无明显界线。真皮下方为皮下组织（3）含有脂肪、血管、淋巴管、神经、汗腺及环层小体等。

1. Section 1: Skin of finger

Materials and methods: Skin of human finger, HE staining.

LPM: Figure 11-1a shows the skin of finger. The skin is composed of epidermis (1) and dermis (2). The epidermis consists of stratified keratinized squamous epithelium and the dermis consists of the connective tissue that supports the epidermis and binds it to the underlying subcutis/hypodermis. The dermis contains two layers: the outermost papillary layer and the deeper reticular layer. The subcutis (3) contains adipose tissue, blood vessels, lymphvessels, nerves, sweat glands and Pacinian corpuscles, et al.

（1）手指皮肤——表皮

高倍镜观察：图 11-1b 显示表皮为角化的复层扁平上皮，由表皮的基底层向表面观察，可见表皮由五层结构组成：基底层（1），由一层立方形或低柱状细胞组成，细胞界限不清。棘层（2），位于基底层的上方，为数层多边形的细胞。颗粒层（3），在多边形细胞的上方，为数层梭形的细胞，呈波纹状起伏。细胞内含有强嗜碱性的深蓝色颗粒，即透明角质颗粒。透明层，一般只能在厚一些的皮肤中看到，为数层细胞质较透明、嗜酸性的扁平细胞组成，没有细胞核和细胞器。角质层（4），在透明层的上方，染色为红色，很厚，由数层角化的扁平细胞组成。

Skin of finger—Epidermis

Materials and methods: Human finger skin, HE staining

HPM: Figure 11-1b shows that the epidermis consists of a stratified keratinized squamous epithelium. From basal layer to surface, the epidermis contains five layers. The Basal Layer (1): The basal layer contains a single layer of cubic or short columnar cells located on the basement membrane where the cell boundaries are unclear. The Spinous Layer (2): The stratum spinosum contains several layers of polyhedral or slightly flattened cells located above the basal layer. The Granular Layer (3): The granular layer consists of 3-5 layers of flattened spindle cells located above the polygonal cells. Their cytoplasm is filled with intensely basophilic dark blue granules named keratohyalin granules. The Stratum Lucidum: The stratum lucidum can be only seen in thick skin. It contains a thin, translucent layer of flattened eosinophilic cells without nuclei and organelles. The Stratum Corneum (4): The stratum corneum consists of several layers of flattened, nonnucleated keratinized cells stained red locating above the stratum lucidum.

（2）手指皮肤——真皮

低倍镜观察：图 11-1c 显示真皮，真皮为表皮下方的致密结缔组织。可以分为两层：乳

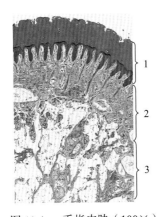

图 11-1a 手指皮肤 (100×)
Fig. 11-1a Skin of finger (100×)

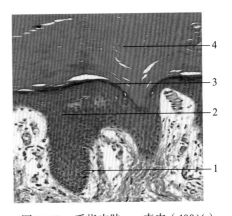

图 11-1b 手指皮肤——表皮 (400×)
Fig. 11-1b Skin—Epidermis of finger (400×)

头层（1）和网织层（2）。乳头层：紧贴表皮下方，较薄，呈乳头状突起嵌入表皮基底面。真皮的乳头层可以分为血管乳头和神经乳头。乳头内可见毛细血管的断面为血管乳头（3）。在神经乳头内可见触觉小体（4）。触觉小体为圆柱形有被囊的神经末梢。中央为横行排列的扁平细胞，表面包有结缔组织被囊，其长轴与皮肤表面垂直，感受触觉。网织层：位于乳头层的下方，较厚，由较粗大的胶原纤维和弹性纤维交织而成。此层内有血管、淋巴管和神经束。深部可见环层小体（图 11-1d）。

Skin of finger—Dermis

LPM: Figure 11-1c shows dermis layer, composed by dense connective tissue and locates beneath the layer of epidermis. The dermis contains two layers with indistinct boundaries: papillary layer (1) and reticular layer (2). The papillary layer, which is close to the lower part of the epidermis, is thinner and has papillary processes embedded in the base of the epidermis. The papillary layer of dermis can be divided into vascular papilla and nerve papilla. The vessel papilla (3) is rich in capillary. Tactile corpuscles (4) can be seen in the nerve papilla. Tactile corpuscles are cylindrical nerve endings with tunic. There are horizontal flat cells in the center and connective tissue capsules on the surface. The long axis of the tactile corpuscle is perpendicular to the surface of the skin.

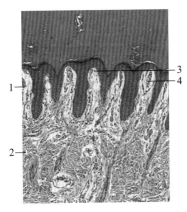

图 11-1c 手指皮肤——真皮 (100×)
Fig. 11-1c Skin of finger—Dermis (100×)

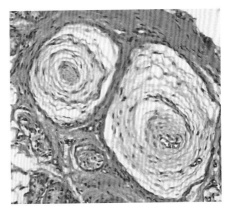

图 11-1d 环层小体 (400×)
Fig. 11-1d Pacinian corpuscle (400×)

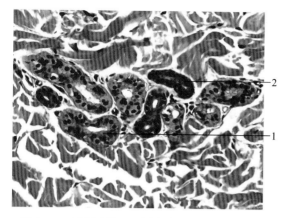

图 11-1e　手指皮肤——汗腺腺泡和导管（400×）

Fig. 11-1e　Ducts and acini of sweat gland in finger skin (400×)

Tactile corpuscles receive tactile sense. The reticular layer: the reticular layer is thicker, composed of irregular dense connective tissue, and contains more fibers, blood vessels, lymphatics and nerves. Pacinian corpuscles (Figure 11-1d) can be also seen in the deep of the reticular layer.

（3）手指皮肤——皮下组织

皮下组织位于真皮层的下方（图 11-1a），含有脂肪组织，较大的血管，淋巴管，神经束，汗腺的导管部和分泌部（图 11-1e）以及环层小体（图 11-1d）。

手指皮肤——环层小体

图 11-1d 显示环层小体为圆形或椭圆形有被囊的神经末梢，中央为同心圆状排列的扁平细胞，表面包有结缔组织被囊。感受压觉。

Skin of finger-dermis—Subcutis layer

The subcutis layer (Figure 11-1a) locate under dermis layer containing adipose tissue, blood vessels, nerves, sweat glands (Figure 11-1e) and Pacinian corpuscles (Figure 11-1d).

Skin of finger—Pacinian corpuscles

Figure 11-1d shows that pacinian corpuscles are annular or elliptic nerve endings with tunic. The flattened cells lie in the center with connective tissue capsules on the surface. Pacinian corpuscles can apperceive touch or pressure as well as vibration and tension.

手指皮肤——汗腺

图 11-1e 显示汗腺，汗腺属于外分泌腺，由腺泡（1）和导管（2）两部分组成：分泌部由单层低柱状或立方形上皮细胞围成腺泡。导管由 2～3 层低柱状上皮细胞组成，管径较小，着色较深。

Skin of finger—sweat gland

Figure 11-1e shows sweat gland, which belongs to the exocrine glands, and contains the secretory portions (1) and ducts (2). The secretory part is lightly-stained than the duct is and has stratified cuboidal epithelial cells. The duct consists of 2-3 layers of short columnar epithelial cells with darker staining and the diameter of duct is small.

❷ 切片 2：人背部皮肤

材料与方法：人背部皮肤，HE 染色。

低倍镜观察：图 11-2a 显示人背部皮肤的表皮较薄（1），角质层也较薄，上皮表面凹凸不平。真皮较厚，由致密结缔组织组成，其内分布有汗腺（2）毛囊（3），皮脂腺（4）及立毛肌。

2. Section 2: Human dorsal skin

Materials and methods: Human dorsal skin, HE staining.

LPM: Figure 11-2a shows that human dorsal skin. The epidermis of dorsal skin is thinner

(1), the stratum corneum is also thinner with uneven surface. The dermis of dorsal skin is thicker composed of dense connective tissue and a few of sweat glands (2), hair follicles (3), sebaceous glands (4) and arrector pili muscle.

人背部皮肤——表皮

高倍镜观察：图 11-2b 显示背皮表皮的结构。图中显示基底层（1）、棘层（2）颗粒层（3）及角质层（4）。细胞之间常夹有黑色素细胞。

Human dorsal skin—Epidermis

HPM: Figure 11-2b shows the structure of the epidermis of dorsal skin. The figure shows basal layer cells (1), spinous layer cells (2) granular layer cells (3) and cornified layer cells (4).There are many melanin granules in the basal layer cells.

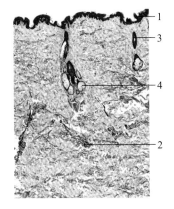 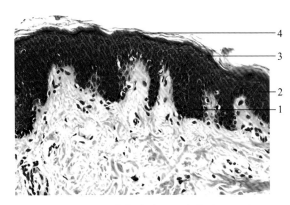

图 11-2a　人背部皮肤（100×）　　　　图 11-2b　人背部皮肤——表皮（400×）

Fig. 11-2a　Human dorsal skin（100×）　　Fig. 11-2b　Human dorsal skin—Epidermis（400×）

❸ 切片 3：人头皮

材料与方法：人头皮，HE 染色。

低倍镜观察：图 11-3a 显示，人头皮的表皮为角化的复层扁平上皮，较薄，角质层也较薄，毛伸出皮肤表面的部分为毛干（1），在皮肤内的部分为毛根（2）。表皮下陷部位形成毛囊（3）。真皮较薄，由致密结缔组织组成，其内分布许多皮脂腺（4）、立毛肌（5）、汗腺（6），及毛囊。皮下组织含有大量的脂肪组织，毛囊，毛球（7）和汗腺。

3. Section3: Human scalp

Materials and methods: Human scalp, HE staining.

LPM: Figure 11-3a shows: The epidermis of scalp is thinly keratinized stratified squamous epithelium. The part of hair extending above the skin surface is the hair shaft (1), and the part imbedding into the skin is the hair root (2). The epidermis invaginate down to form hair follicles (3). The dermis is thinner and consists of dense connective tissue. There are many

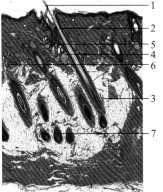

图 11-3a　头皮（100×）

Fig. 11-3a　Scalp（100×）

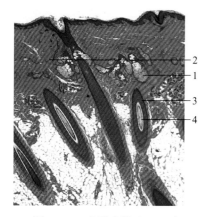

图 11-3b 毛及毛囊（200×）

Fig. 11-3b Hair and hair follicle (200×)

sebaceous glands (4), arrector pili muscle (5), sweat glands (6), and hair follicles in dermis. The subcutis layer contains a lot of adipose tissue, hair follicles, hair bulbs (7) and sweat glands.

人头皮——附属结构

高倍镜观察：图 11-3b 显示，皮脂腺（1）一般位于真皮层中，分泌部由一个或几个囊状腺泡构成，导管由复层扁平上皮组成，通常开口于毛囊的上部。立毛肌（2）是可以控制毛发的平滑肌，一端连接毛囊中侧部位的结缔组织，另一端与皮肤真皮相连。毛囊（3）为包裹的毛根（4）外面的管状上皮鞘。

Human scalp—skin appendages

HPM: The Figure 11-3b shows that sebaceous gland (1) are embedded in the dermis, which secretory portion consists of one or more cystic acinus and ducts compose of stratified squamous epithelium, usually opening at the top of hair follicle. Arrector pili muscle (2) is smooth muscle that controls hair. One end of the arrector pili muscle connects to the connective tissue in the middle of the hair follicle, and the other end directly connects to the dermis of skin. Hair follicle (3) is a tubular epithelium sheath which was packaged by glass membrane and connective tissue sheath, wrapping outside of the hair root (4).

【作业】

绘图描述触觉小体和环层小体的结构。

【Assignment】

Try to describe the structure of Meissner corpuscles and Pacinian corpuscles.

【思考题】

1. 描述毛发的结构特点。
2. 描述指皮和背皮的结构区别。

【Questions】

1. Try to describe the structure characteristics of hair.
2. Try to describe the structural differences between the skin of finger and dorsal skin.

【临床与科研联系英文阅读材料】
【English Reading Material for Correlations with Clinic and Scientific Research】

The skin is the largest organ of human body. It is the first physical defensive line to resist external damage. Skin participates in the body's physiological activities and makes the body in tune with the natural environment. The abnormal condition of the body can also be reflected on the surface of the skin. The skin disease is one of the frequently occurring diseases, including leprosy, scabies, fungus and bacterial skin infections etc. In medicine, skin disease is a common disease, which can affect human's health. The morbidity of skin disease is very high. Although most of the skin diseases do not affect life expectancy, there are serious skin diseases posing huge threat to human life.

（祁丽花）

第12章 内分泌系统

Chapter 12 Endocrine System

【实习内容】Contents of Observation

 切片 Sections

观察切片	Observation Sections
1. 甲状腺和甲状旁腺	1. Thyroid and parathyroid gland
2. 肾上腺	2. Adrenal gland
3. 垂体	3. Pituitary

【目的要求】

1. 掌握垂体的分部、组成细胞及其功能。
2. 掌握甲状腺的结构特点，注意区分静止期与活动期结构特点的不同。
3. 熟悉甲状旁腺的结构特征。
4. 掌握肾上腺的组成及细胞功能。

【Objective】

1. To master the cellular compositions of pituitary gland and their functions respectively.

2. To master the structure of thyroid and compare the structure differences between resting and activity stage of thyroid.

3. To be familiar with the structure of parathyroid gland.

4. To master the compositions and cellular function of adrenal gland.

【观察标本】
【Observation Sections】

1 切片 1: 甲状腺和甲状旁腺

材料与方法: 猫甲状腺与甲状旁腺, HE 染色。

低倍镜观察: 图 12-1a 显示甲状腺 (A) 及其背侧的甲状旁腺 (B)。两者的表面为结缔组织构成的被膜 (1)。甲状腺部分可见大小不等的滤泡 (2), 滤泡腔内有粉红色的胶状物质, 即甲状腺球蛋白 (3)。甲状旁腺部分则染色较深, 细胞排列成团索状。

1. Section 1: Thyroid and Parathyroid Gland

Material and methods: Thyroid and parathyroid gland of the cat, paraffin embedding, HE staining.

LPM: Figure 12-1a shows the thyroid (A) and its dorsal parathyroid gland (B). The surface of both thyroid and parathyroid gland is surrounded by connective tissue capsule (1). The thyroid consists of variable sized follicles (2) with pink colloid, i.e. thyroglobulin (3). The parathyroid gland stains deeply and cells are arranged in clusters.

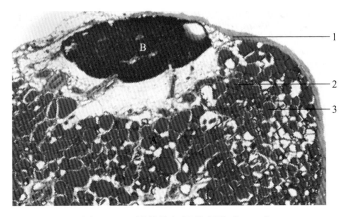

图 12-1a　甲状腺与甲状旁腺 (25×)

Fig. 12-1a　Thyroid and parathyroid (25×)

(1) 甲状腺

低倍镜观察: 图 12-1b 显示甲状腺由大小不等的甲状腺滤泡 (1) 构成。滤泡内为胶状物 (2)。滤泡间结缔组织内可见血管 (3)。

高倍镜观察: 图 12-1c 显示甲状腺滤泡上皮为单层立方 (1) 或柱状上皮 (甲状腺滤泡功能活跃时)。细胞核圆形, 染色较深。滤泡腔内充满粉红色胶状物 (2)。在滤泡之间或滤泡上皮细胞之间, 可见滤泡旁细胞 (3), 该细胞体积较大, 单个或团状存在, 细胞质染色较浅。细胞核较大、呈圆形, 染色也较浅。

(1) Thyroid

LPM: Figure 12-1b shows that the thyroid consists of varied sized follicles (1). The follicle cavities contain colloids (2). The capillaries (3) can be observed in connective tissues among follicles.

HPM: Figure 12-1c shows thyroid follicles with a simple cuboidal epithelium (1) or simple columnar epithelium (when undergoing active colloid resorption). The follicular cells have a round, and darkly stained nuclei. The follicular cavity contains pink colloid (2). The parafollicular cells (3) distribute singly or in small clumps among the interfollicular position with large size and clear, lightly stained cytoplasm.

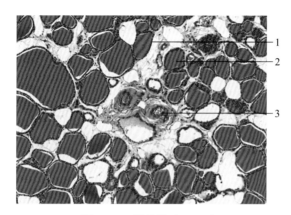

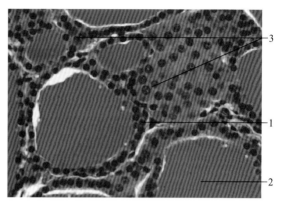

图 12-1b　甲状腺（100×）

Fig. 12-1b　Thyroid (100×)

图 12-1c　甲状腺（400×）

Fig. 12-1c　Thyroid (400×)

（2）甲状旁腺

低倍镜观察：图 12-1d 显示甲状旁腺。其表面为薄层结缔组织被膜（1），实质细胞（2）排列成团、索状。索状结缔组织间可见毛细血管（3）。

高倍镜观察：图 12-1e 显示甲状旁腺的组成细胞主要为主细胞和嗜酸性细胞。主细胞（1）数量多、排列成索状。嗜酸性细胞（2）较大、嗜酸性，非规则排列，单独或数个聚集成团存在。

(2) Parathyroid gland

LPM: Figure 12-1d shows the parathyroid gland. Its surface is covered by delicate connective tissue capsule (1). The Parenchymal cells (2) are arrange in cluster s or, cords. The capillaries (3) are among funicular connective tissue in the stroma.

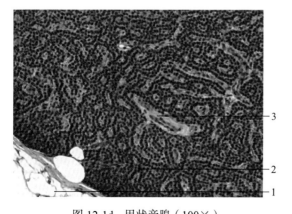

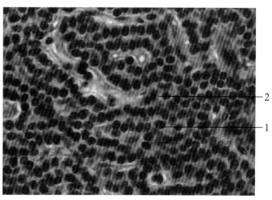

图 12-1d　甲状旁腺（100×）

Fig. 12-1d　Parathyroid gland (100×)

图 12-1e　甲状旁腺（400×）

Fig. 12-1e　Parathyroid gland (400×)

HPM: Figure 12-1e shows that parathyroid gland consists of chief cells and eosinophil cells. Chief cells (1) are numerous and are arranged in cords; eosinophil (2) are larger, more acidophilic cells, which are irregularly distributed and occur singly or in clumps.

② 切片 2：肾上腺

材料与方法：猫肾上腺，HE 染色。

低倍镜观察：

图 12-2a 显示肾上腺全层结构。外部的被膜（1）为致密的结缔组织膜。皮质分为球状带（2）、束状带（3）和网状带（4）三个不同的区带，细胞呈团状或索状，垂直于被膜排列。髓质（5）位于内侧，细胞呈不规则网状排列，内含毛细血管和大的静脉窦（6）。

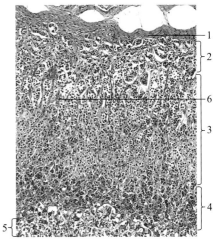

图 12-2a　肾上腺（100×）

Fig. 12-2a　Adrenal gland（100×）

2. Section 2: Adrenal Gland

Materials and methods: Adrenal gland of the cat, paraffin embedding, HE staining.

LPM: Figure 12-2a shows the full adrenal parenchyma layers. The outer capsule (1) is made of dense fibrous connective tissue. The cortex has three distinct zones, zona glomerulosa (ZG, 2), zona fasciculata (ZF, 3), zona reticularis (ZR, 4), with cells arranged in clumps or cords perpendicular to the capsule. The inner medulla (5) has an irregular network of cells in close association with abundant capillaries and large venous sinusoids (6).

高倍镜观察：

1）球状带（图 12-2b）：紧靠被膜，约占皮质厚度的 15%。细胞（1）呈低柱状或立方形，排列成球形细胞团，核小而圆，染色深。基质中可见毛细血管（2）。

2）束状带（图 12-2c）：占皮质厚度 65%～80%，细胞（1）体积大，为圆形或多边形。由于类脂质被溶之故，胞质多呈空泡状（2），核大而圆，胞质染色浅。细胞排列成束，细胞索之间可见血窦（3）。

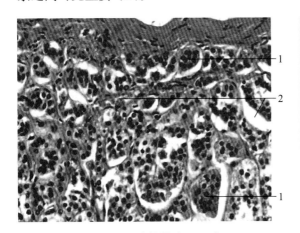

图 12-2b　球状带（200×）

Fig. 12-2b　Zona glomerulosa（200×）

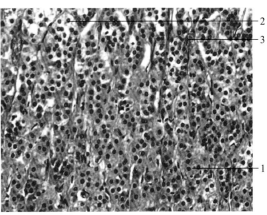

图 12-2c　束状带（200×）

Fig. 12-2c　Zona fasciculata（200×）

HPM:

1) ZG: Figure 12-2b, the zona glomerulosa, immediately inside the capsule and comprising about 15% of the cortex, consists of closely packed, rounded or arched cords of columnar, or cubic cells (1), with darkly stained nuclei, and unclear cellular boundaries. The capillaries (2) can be observed in stroma.

2) ZF: Figure 12-2c, zona fasciculata, occupies 65% to 80% of the cortex and consists of long cords of large polyhedral cells (1) with vacuolar cytoplasm, larger and round nuclei. The cells are filled with lipid droplets and appear vacuolated (2). The sinusoids (3) can be observed between cellular cords.

3）网状带（图 12-2d）：约占皮质厚度的 10%，细胞（1）体积较小，排列成不规则的条索状，交织成网，细胞索间有丰富的血窦（2）。染色较束状带（3）细胞深，是由于脂滴含量相对较少的缘故。网状带内侧是髓质（4）。

4）髓质（图 12-2e）：嗜铬细胞（1）排列成索状，胞体较大，形态不一，胞质清明，但分界不清，核大而圆，着色较浅，细胞索间可见毛细血管（2）。有的切片中可见到交感神经节细胞（3）。图中（4）为皮质的网状带细胞。

3) ZR: Figure 12-2d, zona reticularis comprises about 10% of the cortex and consists of smaller cells (1) in a network of irregular cords interspersed with wide capillaries (2). The cells are round, and small, with round nuclei and deeply stained cytoplasm than those of the zona fasciculate (3) because they contain fewer lipid. Medial to the zona reticularis is the medulla (4).

4) Medulla: Figure 12-2e shows that the chromaffin cells (1) arranged in irregular cords with clear cytoplasm, but unclear cellular boundaries. The nuclei are large and round, lightly stained. There are sinusoidal capillaries (3) between adjacent cords and a few parasympathetic ganglion cells (4) are present. The cells of zona reticularis show as (4).

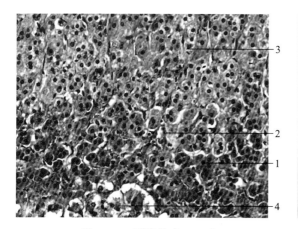

图 12-2d　网状带（200×）

Fig. 12-2d　Zona reticularis (200×)

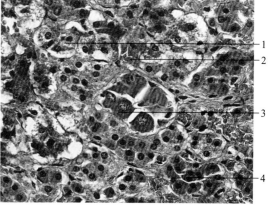

图 12-2e　肾上腺髓质（400×）

Fig. 12-2e　Medulla of adrenal gland (400×)

❸ 切片 3：垂体

材料与方法：人脑垂体，HE 染色。

低倍镜观察：图 12-3a 显示垂体横断面的三个部分：腺垂体远侧部（A），染色较深；腺垂体中间部（B），含有许多充满胶质的囊；以及神经垂体的神经部（C），染色较浅。

3. Section 3: Pituitary

Materials and methods: pituitary gland of human, paraffin embedding, HE staining.

LPM: Figure 12-3a shows the three parts in cross section of pituitary: the pars distalis of adenohypophysis (A) with deeper staining, the pars intermedia of adenohypophysis (B) with numerous colloid-filled cysts, and pars nervosa of neurohypophysis (C) with pale staining.

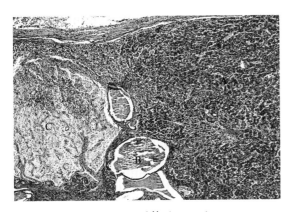

图 12-3a　垂体（400×）

Fig. 12-3a　Pituitary（400×）

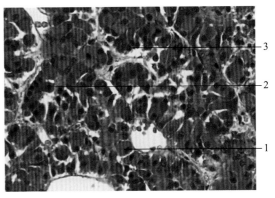

图 12-3b　腺垂体远侧部（400×）

Fig. 12-3b　Pars distalis of adenohypophysis（400×）

高倍镜观察：

（1）图 12-3b 显示远侧部细胞呈团索状排列，细胞之间有结缔组织和血窦，可以观察到染成红色的嗜酸性细胞（1）、染成蓝色的嗜碱性细胞（2）以及染色较浅的嫌色细胞（3）。

（2）图 12-3c 显示腺垂体中间部的细胞排列成滤泡样，腔内有胶状物（1），也有一些细胞排列成团索样结构（2）。

（3）图 12-3d 显示神经垂体的神经部含有许多无髓鞘神经纤维（1），梭形多突的垂体细胞（2）和丰富的毛细血管（3），镜下有时可见大小不等的嗜酸性团块，即赫令体（4），是轴突内分泌颗粒大量聚集所成的结构。

HPM:

(1) Figure 12-3b shows the cells of pars distalis of adenohypophysis arranged in cords. There

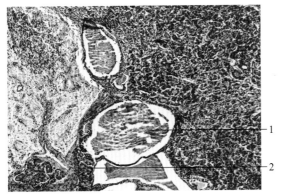

图 12-3c　垂体中间部（100×）

Fig. 12-3c　Pars intermedia of adenohypophysis（100×）

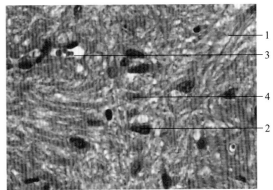

图 12-3d　神经垂体神经部（400×）

Fig. 12-3d　Pars nervosa of neurohypophysis（400×）

are connective tissues and sinusoids. The acidophiles (1) have pink-staining cytoplasm; basophils (2) have blue-staining cytoplasm, and chromophobes (3) have pale staining cytoplasm.

(2) Figure 12-3c shows the cells of pars intermedia of adenohypophysis arranged in follicles, with colloids in cavities. Some cells are arranged in cords.

(3) Figure 12-3d shows that the pars nervosa of neurohypophysis contain numerous unmyelinated nerve fiber (1), spindle-shaped pituicytes (2), and capillaries (3). Herring body (4), a structure composed of axon endocrine particles, which shows as eosinophilic clumps of varying size under LM.

【思考题】

1. 试述甲状腺滤泡上皮细胞的结构和功能。
2. 试述肾上腺皮质、髓质的结构及分泌的激素。
3. 试述腺垂体远侧部细胞光镜下的结构及功能。
4. 试述神经垂体的组成及其与下丘脑的关系。
5. 试述垂体门脉系统的组成及其功能意义。

【Questions】

1. Please describe the structure and function of thyroid follicular epithelium.

2. Please describe the structure of cortex and medulla of adrenal gland, and its secretion of hormones.

3. Please describe the structure and function of pars distalis of adenohypophysis under light microscopy.

4. Please describe the composition of pars nervosa of neurohypophysis, its relationship with hypothalamus.

5. Please describe the composition of pituitary portal system and its function.

【临床与科研联系英文阅读材料】 【English Reading Material for Correlations with Clinic and Scientific Research】

Graves disease is characterized by hyperplasia of the follicular cells, increasing the size of thyroid gland two to three times above normal. Thyroid hormone production is also greatly increased, many times of normal (hyperthyroidism). Other symptoms include excess sweating, anxiety, exophthalmos (protrusion of the eyeballs), diarrhea, hair loss et cetera. Although Graves disease may develop from several causes, the most common agent is the binding of autoimmune immunoglobulin G (IgG) antibodies to TSH receptors, which stimulates thyroid follicular cells. Insufficient dietary intake of iodine causes the thyroid gland to enlarge, a condition called simple goiter. Goiter usually is not associated with hyperthyroidism or hypothyroidism. This condition can be treated with supplementation of iodine in the diet.

（王大亮）

第13章 消化管

Chapter 13 Digestive Tract

【实习内容】Contents of Observation

切片　Sections

观察切片	Observation Sections
1. 舌	1. Lingua
2. 食管	2. Esophagus
3. 胃底	3. Stomach fundus
4. 胃幽门和十二指肠	4. Stomach pylorus and duodenum
5. 空肠	5. Jejunum
6. 回肠	6. Ileum
7. 结肠	7. Colon
8. 阑尾	8. Appendix

【目的要求】

1. 掌握消化管壁的微细结构，正确区分各段。
2. 掌握食管壁的特征性结构。
3. 掌握胃黏膜的特征性结构。
4. 掌握小肠黏膜的特征性结构，正确区分十二指肠、空肠和回肠。
5. 掌握结肠的结构。
6. 了解舌乳头的形态结构。

【 Objective 】

1. To master microscopic structure of the wall of digestive tract，and correctly identify different organs in the digestive tract.

2. To master characteristic structure of esophagus.

3. To master characteristic structure of stomach mucosa.

4. To master characteristic structure of small intestinal mucosa, and correctly identify duodenum, jejunum and ileum.

5. To master morphological features of colon.

6. To know morphological structure of lingual papilla.

【 观察切片 】
【 Observation Sections 】

1 切片1：舌

材料与方法：人或动物舌，HE 染色。

低倍镜观察：图 13-1a 显示舌黏膜由复层扁平上皮与固有层组成，可见舌乳头（1）。舌乳头周围有环沟，沟两侧的上皮内有多个淡染的卵圆形小体，为味蕾（2）；固有层中有浆液性腺（3），导管（4）开口于沟底。

高倍镜观察：图 13-1b 显示环沟两侧上皮内味蕾（1）的形态结构。味蕾顶端有味孔（2），味蕾中长梭形的细胞为味细胞（3），味蕾深部呈锥体形的细胞是基细胞（4）。

1. Section 1: Lingua

Materials and methods: Human or animal lingua, HE staining.

LPM: Figure 13-1a shows that the mucosa of the tongue consists of stratified squamous epithelium and lamina propria. Papillae (1) can be seen, which surrounded by deep moats. The light-staining oval taste buds (2) are embedded in the epithelium lining the side wall of the papillae. The lingual salivary glands (3) are located in the lamina propria. Ducts (4) of the glands empty a serous

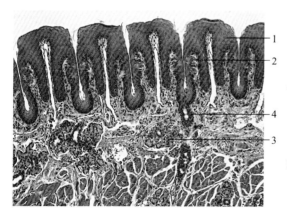

图 13-1a　舌（100×）

Fig. 13-1a　Lingua (100×)

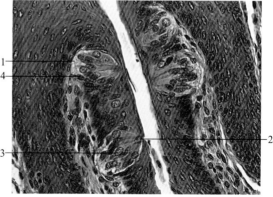

图 13-1b　味蕾（400×）

Fig. 13-1b　Taste buds (400×)

secretion into the base of the moat.

HPM: Figure 13-1b shows morphological structure of the taste buds (1) in the epithelium lining the side wall of the papillae. On the apical part of the taste bud is a small opening-the taste pore (2). In the taste bud, the spindle-like tall cells are the taste cells (3), while the small pyramidal cells are the basal cells (4) located near the base of the taste bud.

❷ 切片 2：食管

材料与方法：人食管，HE 染色。

低倍镜观察：图 13-2 显示黏膜上皮为未角化的复层扁平上皮（1）。固有层（2）浅染，为疏松结缔组织，可见淋巴组织、小血管及食管腺导管。黏膜肌层（3）为一层纵行平滑肌束的横断面。黏膜下层由疏松结缔组织构成，可见血管和黏液性的食管腺（4）。肌层（5）分内环行（肌纤维纵切面）、外纵行（横切面）两层，其间可见肌间神经丛。肌纤维的类型因取材部位不同而异，可以是平滑肌或骨骼肌。外膜：为纤维膜。

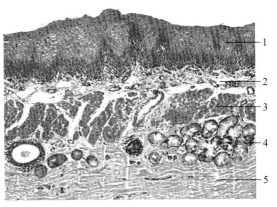

图 13-2　食管（100×）
Fig. 13-2　Esophagus (100×)

2. Section 2: Esophagus

Materials and methods: Human esophagus, HE staining.

LPM: Figure 13-2 shows that the mucous epithelium is non-keratinized stratified squamous epithelium (1). The lamina propria (2) is light-staining and consists of fine connective tissue with lymphatic tissue, small blood vessels and the ducts of esophageal glands. The muscularis mucosae (3) is formed by longitudinally-arranged smooth muscle fibers. The submucosa is made up by loose connective tissue, where the blood vessels and the mucous esophageal glands (4) are present. The muscularis externa (5) is relatively thick, with an outer longitudinal and an inner circular layer of muscle. The myenteric nerve plexus can be seen between muscle layers. In the upper segment of the esophagus, the muscularis externa contains skeletal muscle. In the middle segment, it contains both skeletal and smooth muscle. While in the lower segment, it contains smooth muscle. Determine which segment the section was taken from according to the type of muscle you find here. The adventitia is a fibrous coat of loose connective tissue.

❸ 切片 3：胃底

材料与方法：人或动物胃底，HE 染色。

低倍镜观察：图 13-3a 显示胃底分为 4 层，黏膜（1）、黏膜下层（2）、肌层（3）和外膜（4）。黏膜由上皮、固有层和黏膜肌层构成。黏膜下层为较致密的结缔组织。肌层由内斜、中环和外纵的平滑肌组成。外膜为浆膜，由少量疏松结缔组织和间皮构成。图 13-3b 显示胃黏膜上皮（1）为单层柱状，由表面黏液细胞组成，无杯状细胞。上皮内陷形成胃小凹（2）。固有层可见密集的胃底腺（3），胃底腺由 5 种细胞组成：主细胞、壁细胞、颈黏液细胞、内分泌细胞和干细胞，腺体间有少量结缔组织和散在的平滑肌纤维。黏膜肌层（4）为薄层平滑肌。黏膜下层为较致密的结缔组织，内含血管、神经和淋巴管，可见黏膜下神经丛。

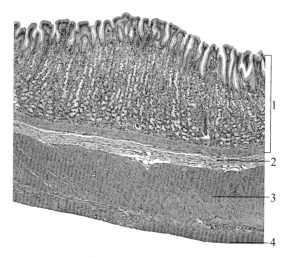

图 13-3a　胃底（40×）

Fig. 13-3a　Stomach fundus (40×)

3. Section 3: Stomach fundus

Materials and methods: Human or animal stomach fundus, HE staining.

LPM: Figure 13-3a shows four layers of stomach fundus: mucosa (1), submucosa (2), muscularis propria (3) and adventitia (4). The mucosa consists of epithelium, lamina propria and muscularis mucosa. The submucosa is made up by the dense connective tissue. The muscularis propria is relatively thick, with three layers of smooth muscle, inner oblique, middle circular and outer longitudinal layers. Adventitaia is the serosa, which consists of a thin layer of loose connective tissue and mesothelium. Figure 13-3b shows that the gastric mucosa epithelium (1) is simple columnar epithelium, which is composed of surface mucous cells, but no goblet cells. The epithelium invaginates to form gastric pits (2). The lamina propria is filled with many tubular fundic glands (3). A few smooth muscle cells and scattered connective tissue are present between the fundic glands. The fundic gland consists of five types of cells: chief cell, parietal cell, mucous neck cell, endocrine cell and stem cell. The muscularis mucosae (4) is a thin smooth muscle coat. The submucosa is made up by the dense connective tissue containing small blood vessels, nerves and lymphatic vessels. The submucosal plexus can be seen in the submucosa.

高倍镜观察：图 13-3c 显示胃底腺的主细胞和壁细胞，主细胞（1）主要分布于胃底腺的下半部。细胞小，呈柱状，核圆，位于基底部；基部胞质呈强嗜碱性，着紫蓝色，顶部充满红色酶原颗粒，在普通固定染色标本上，此颗粒多溶解而呈泡沫状，故着色浅淡。壁细胞（2）在胃底腺的上半部较多。胞体呈圆形或圆锥形，较大；核圆居中，胞质嗜酸性，呈红色。

HPM: Figure 13-3c shows that the chief cells are mainly found in the lower half of the fundic

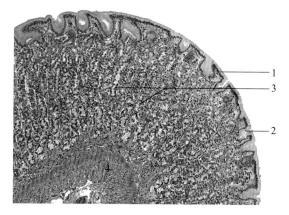

图 13-3b　胃底（100×）

Fig. 13-3b　Stomach fundus (100×)

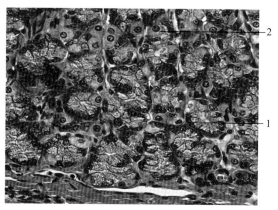

图 13-3c　胃底腺（400×）

Fig. 13-3c　Fundic gland (400×)

glands. Chief cell (1) is columnar in shape. The round nucleus lies in the base of the cell. The basal cytoplasm is strong basophilic and stained purple-blue. There are many red zymogen granules in the apical region of the cytoplasm. These granules dissolve during routine specimen fixation, thus the apical cytoplasm stains lightly. The parietal cells (2) mainly distribute in the upper part of the fundic glands. They are large, spherical or pyramidal in shape. The cytoplasm is deeply acidophilic and stains red. The nucleus is central-placed. Sometimes, two nuclei can be found in one cell.

❹ 切片 4：胃幽门和十二指肠

材料与方法：人或动物胃幽门和十二指肠连接处，HE 染色。

低倍镜观察：图 13-4a 显示幽门部（1）和十二指肠（2）。幽门部可见胃小凹（3），且较胃底部深，固有层中有幽门腺（4），其余各层与胃底部相似。十二指肠黏膜有许多由单层柱状上皮和固有层突向肠腔形成的绒毛（5），呈叶状。可见到绒毛的不同切面。绒毛根部以下的固有层中有许多不同断面的小肠腺（6），可有孤立淋巴小结。图 13-4b 显示黏膜（1）、黏膜下层（2）、肌层（3）和外膜（4）。黏膜下层为疏松结缔组织，可见大量黏液性十二指肠腺（5），是十二指肠的特征。肌层（3）由内环行和外纵行两层平滑肌组成，可见肌间神经丛。外膜多为浆膜。

4. Section 4: Stomach pylorus and duodenum

Materials and methods: Human or animal, the junction between stomach pylorus and duodenum, HE staining.

LPM: Figure 13-4a shows stomach pylorus (1) and duodenum (2). In stomach pylorus, The gastric pits (3) are deeper than those in the stomach fundus. The lamina propria contains pyloric glands (4). Other structural features of the stomach pylorus are similar to those of the stomach fundus. There are many leafy-looking intestinal villus (5) which are composed of simple columnar epithelium and lamina propria protruding into the lumen of the duodenum. Beneath the base of the villi, the lamina propria contains small intestinal glands (6) and solitary lymphoid aggregates. Figure 13-4b demonstrates mucosa (1), submucosa (2), muscularis (3) and adventitia (4). The submucosa is composed of loose

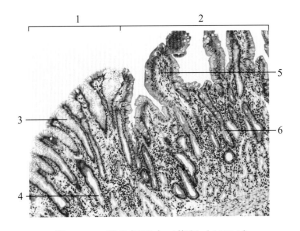

图 13-4a　胃幽门和十二指肠（100×）

Fig. 13-4a　Stomach pylorus and duodenum（100×）

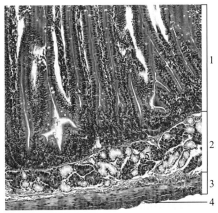

图 13-4b　十二指肠（100×）

Fig. 13-4b　Duodenum（100×）

connective tissue containing many mucous duodenal glands, Brunner's glands (5), which are unique in the duodenum. The muscularis is composed of two layers of smooth muscles, the inner circular and the outer longitudinal layers. The myenteric nerve plexus can be seen. Most parts of adventitia in the duodenum are serosa, meaning the connective tissue is lined by mesothelium.

❺ 切片 5：空肠

材料与方法：人或动物空肠，HE 染色。

低倍镜观察：图 13-5a 显示空肠壁具有与十二指肠相似的 4 层结构。可见不同切面的肠绒毛（1）；固有层中有孤立淋巴小结（2）；黏膜下层无腺体；外膜为浆膜。

高倍镜观察：图 13-5b，可见小肠绒毛上皮吸收细胞游离缘的纹状缘（1）更清晰，杯状细胞增多。绒毛中轴结缔组织内有毛细血管（2）、中央乳糜管（3）及散在的平滑肌（4）。图 13-5c 显示绒毛（1）和小肠腺（2）。小肠腺由 5 种细胞构成，其中的吸收细胞（3）、杯状细胞（4）和帕内特细胞（5）易辨认。小肠腺中的吸收细胞和杯状细胞形态与绒毛上皮中的相似，小肠腺底部的帕内特细胞常三五成群，细胞呈锥体形，胞质顶部充满粗大的染成红色的嗜酸性颗粒。内分泌细胞和干细胞不易分辨。

5. Section 5: Jejunum

Materials and methods: Human or animal jejunum, HE staining.

LPM: Figure 13-5a shows that the wall of the jejunum also contains 4 layers similar to those of the duodenum. The different sectioning planes of intestinal villus (1) can be seen. There are solitary lymphoid aggregates (2) in the lamina propria. There is no gland in the submucosa. The adventitia is covered by serosa.

HPM: Figure 13-5b shows that the striated border (1) covering the free surface of the absorptive cells is more prominent. The numbers of goblet cells increase. In the center of the villus, there are capillaries (2), a central lacteal (3), and scattered smooth muscle cells (4). Figure 13-5c shows intestinal villi (1) and small intestinal glands (2). Small intestinal gland consists of 5 type of cells, where absorptive cells (3), goblet cells (4), and Paneth cells (5) can be identified, stem cells and endocrine cells are not easily recognizable.

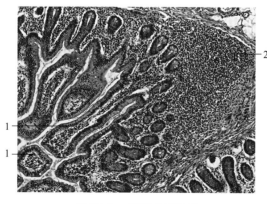

图 13-5a　空肠（100×）
Fig. 13-5a　Jejunum (100×)

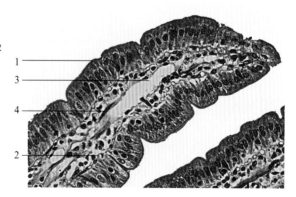

图 13-5b　空肠绒毛（400×）
Fig. 13-5b　Jejunum villus (400×)

❻ 切片6：回肠

材料与方法：人或动物回肠，HE 染色。

低倍镜观察：回肠壁也有典型的 4 层结构，但皱襞较低，绒毛较短而稀疏。图 13-6 显示不同切面的绒毛（1），上皮内的杯状细胞较多，固有层中可见多个淋巴小结聚集形成的集合淋巴小结（2），可穿过黏膜肌层抵达黏膜下层。

高倍镜观察：与空肠相似。

6. Section 6: Ileum

Materials and methods: Human or animal ileum, HE staining.

LPM: The four layers of the ileum wall can be recognized. The plicae are lower and the intestinal villi becomes shorter and sparse. Figure 13-6 shows different sectioning planes of the intestinal villi (1). There are more goblet cells in the epithelium. In lamina propria, several solitary lymph nodules aggregate and form the Peyer's patches (2), which can penetrate the muscularis mucosae and extend into the submucosa.

HPM: The structural features of the ileum are similar to those of the jejunum.

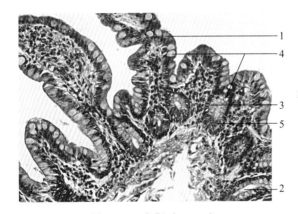

图 13-5c　空肠（400×）

Fig. 13-5c　Jejunum（400×）

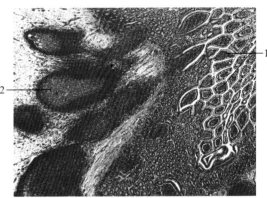

图 13-6　回肠（40×）

Fig. 13-6　Ileum（40×）

❼ 切片7：结肠

材料与方法：人或动物结肠，HE 染色。

低倍镜观察：与小肠壁结构相比，结肠黏膜面平坦，无绒毛。图 13-7a 显示固有层中有密集的大肠腺（1），较小肠腺粗而长，杯状细胞明显多于小肠腺。有的可见孤立淋巴小结。外纵行肌（2）局部增厚形成三条结肠带。外膜为浆膜。图 13-7b 显示结肠上皮为单层柱状，上皮和大肠腺内可见大量的杯状细胞（1）。大肠腺（2）为单管状腺，由吸收细胞、杯状细胞、干细胞和内分泌细胞构成，左半结肠基本上没有帕内特细胞。

7. Section 7: Colon

Materials and methods: Human or animal colon, HE staining.

LPM: Compared with the small intestine, the colonic mucosa is relatively flat and lacks villus. Figure 13-7a shows that the large intestinal glands (1) are dense thicker and longer than small intestinal glands in the lamina propria. The epithelium contains large numbers of goblet cells.

Sometimes solitary lymphoid nodule can be seen. The outer longitudinal layer of the muscularis (2) is organized into three thick, longitudinal bands. The outer surface is covered by serosa. Figure 13-7b shows that the inner surface of colon is covered by simple columnar epithelium, many goblet cells (1) can be found in the surface epithelium as well as in the large intestinal glands. The large intestinal glands (2) are single tubular glands located in laminar propria, which consist of absorptive cells, goblet cells, stem cells and endocrine cells. There is essentially no Paneth cell in the left colon.

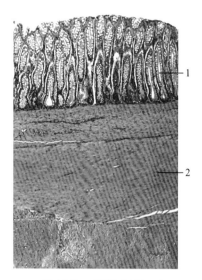

图 13-7a　结肠（100×）
Fig. 13-7a　Colon（100×）

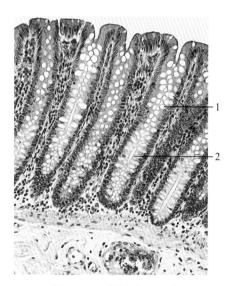

图 13-7b　结肠（200×）
Fig. 13-7b　Colon（200×）

❽ 切片 8：阑尾

材料与方法：人阑尾，HE 染色。

低倍镜观察：图 13-8 显示阑尾黏膜无绒毛，大肠腺（1）少而短，杯状细胞较少；固有层内有极丰富的淋巴组织，多个淋巴小结（2）与弥散淋巴组织连续成层，多深入至黏膜下层，使黏膜肌层不完整；肌层很薄；外膜为浆膜。

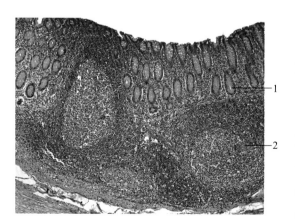

图 13-8　阑尾（100×）
Fig. 13-8　Appendix（100×）

8. Section 8: Appendix

Materials and methods: Human appendix, HE staining.

LPM: Figure 13-8 shows that there is no villus in the mucosa of appendix. The large intestinal glands (1) are shorter and decrease in number, with less goblet cells. The lamina propria contains rich lymphatic tissue. Many lymphatic nodules (2) and diffuse lymphatic tissue form a sheath of lymphoid structure, which penetrate the muscularis mucosae and extend into the submucosa. The muscularis is very thin. The outermost layer is covered by serosa.

【作业】

绘制胃黏膜的高倍镜结构图。

【 Assignment 】

Drawing to describe the morphological structures of gastric mucosa under high power microscopy.

【思考题】

1．消化管管壁由几层组成？其中哪一层变化最明显？
2．食管壁的结构特点是什么？肌层中可能看见哪几种肌纤维？
3．如何区别小肠与胃，小肠与结肠？

【 Questions 】

1. What is the general structure of the wall of the digestive tract? In different parts of the digestive tract, which layer changes most obviously?

2. What are the structural features of esophageal wall? In the muscularis propria, which kinds of muscle fibers can be found?

3. How to distinguish between stomach and small intestine? How to distinguish between small intestine and colon?

【临床与科研联系英文阅读材料】
【 English Reading Material for Correlations with Clinic and Scientific Research 】

Gastric cancer (GC) is the fifth most common malignancy and third leading cause of death from cancer worldwide. There is geographical variation in GC incidence, with Asia being the most common region, with lower rates in USA and Europe. Although incidence has been decreasing in recent decades in Europe, the 5-year survival remains poor (24%). In Japan and Korea, high incidence and historically poor survival rates for gastric cancer have led to the introduction of surveillance program, which has increased 5-year survival to 60%. *Helicobacter pylori* (*H. pylori*), chronic inflammation of the stomach mucosa results in atrophic changes, with loss of structured glandular cells being replaced by intestinal-type epithelium, pyloric-type glands and fibrous tissue. The subsequent gastric atrophy (GA) and intestinal metaplasia (IM) are known premalignant lesions for stomach cancer.

（郭晓霞　尚宏伟）

第14章 消 化 腺

Chapter 14 Digestive Glands

【实习内容】Contents of Observation

切片　Sections

观察切片	Observation Sections
1. 腮腺	1. Parotid gland
2. 舌下腺	2. Sublingual gland
3. 颌下腺	3. Submandibular gland
4. 胰腺	4. Pancreas
5. 猪肝	5. Pork liver
6. 人肝	6. Human liver
7. 胆囊	7. Gall bladder

【目的要求】

1. 掌握浆液性腺泡、黏液性腺泡、混合性腺泡的结构特点。
2. 掌握胰腺的结构特点。
3. 掌握肝的结构特点。

【Objective】

1. To master structural features of serous acinus, mucous acinus, and seromucous acinus.
2. To master morphological features of pancreas.
3. To master morphological features of liver.

【观察切片】
【Observation Sections】

① 切片1：腮腺

材料与方法：人腮腺，HE 染色。

低倍镜观察：图 14-1a 显示腮腺实质被结缔组织分隔成许多小叶，小叶内有大量浆液性腺泡（1）和各级导管的断面。分泌管（又称纹状管）（2）较粗，腔大；闰管（3）细，腔小。结缔组织中有许多脂肪细胞（4）。

高倍镜观察：图 14-1b，腺泡（1）由浆液性细胞构成，胞核圆，位于基部；顶部胞质嗜酸性，基底部胞质嗜碱性。腺泡细胞与基膜（2）之间可见肌上皮细胞（3），其胞核呈长梭形，深染，胞质不易分辨。分泌管（4）较粗，管壁为单层柱状上皮，胞核圆形，近细胞顶部，胞质嗜酸性，基底部可见纵纹。闰管位于腺泡与分泌管之间，腔窄，管壁由单层扁平或立方上皮组成。

1. Section 1: Parotid gland

Materials and methods: Human parotid gland, HE staining.

LPM: Figure 14-1a shows that the connective tissue penetrates into the parenchyma of the gland, and divides the parenchyma into many lobules. In each lobule, there are many serous acini (1) and different types of ducts. The secretory duct (striated duct) (2) is thicker and has a larger lumen. The intercalated duct (3) is thinner and has a smaller lumen. Many adipocytes (4) are seen in connective tissue.

HPM: In Figure 14-1b, the acinus (1) consists of serous cells, with basal located round nucleus. The apical cytoplasm of the cell is acidophilic, while the basal cytoplasm is basophilic. Between the serous cells and the basement membrane (2), myoepithelial cells (3) can be seen. The nuclei are spindle and dark staining. The secretory duct (4) is thicker. The wall of the striated duct is composed of simple columnar epithelium. The epithelial cell nucleus is round and apical located. The cytoplasm is acidophilic. Fine striations can be found at the basal portion of the cell. The intercalated duct leads

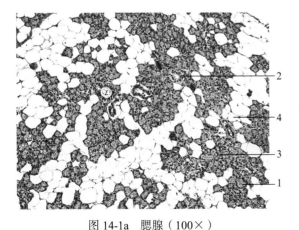

图 14-1a 腮腺（100×）
Fig. 14-1a Parotid gland (100×)

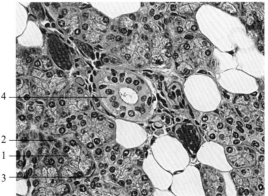

图 14-1b 腮腺（400×）
Fig. 14-1b Parotid gland (400×)

directly from the acinus to a secretory duct. The lumen of the intercalated duct is narrow. The wall of the duct is composed of simple squamous or cuboidal epithelium.

❷ 切片 2：舌下腺

材料与方法：人舌下腺，HE 染色。

低倍镜观察：图 14-2a，结缔组织伸入腺实质将其分隔成许多小叶，小叶内有许多颜色深浅不一的腺泡，颜色深者为浆液性腺泡（1），浅者是黏液性腺泡（2），有的由浆液性和黏液性腺细胞混合形成混合性腺泡（3），但以黏液性腺泡为多。腺泡间及小叶间可见导管（4）的断面。

高倍镜观察：图 14-2b 显示浆液性腺泡（1）：由浆液性细胞组成，胞核圆，位于基部；基部胞质嗜碱性，顶部胞质嗜酸性。黏液性腺泡：由黏液性细胞组成，胞核扁圆，染色深，位于细胞基部；胞质着色浅淡，呈空泡状。混合性腺泡（2）：由浆液性和黏液性细胞混合组成，多数腺泡以黏液性细胞为主，少量的浆液性细胞常聚集于腺泡的一端，在切片中呈半月形，称浆半月（3）。导管（4）：上皮因管径大小而异，小者多为立方或柱状，大者多为高柱状或复层上皮。

2. Section 2: Sublingual gland

Materials and methods: Human sublingual gland, HE staining.

LPM: Figure 14-2a shows that the connective tissue penetrates into the parenchyma of the gland, and divides the parenchyma into many lobules. In the lobule, there are many dark or light staining acini. The dark-staining acini are serous acinus (1), and the light-staining acini are mucous acinus (2). The seromucous acinus (3) contains both serous and mucous cells. In the sublingual gland, most acini are mucous. The ducts (4) can be seen in the lobules or in the interlobular septae.

HPM: In Figure 14-2b, the serous acinus (1) consists of serous cells, with basal located round nucleus. The apical cytoplasm of the cell is acidophilic, while the basal cytoplasm is basophilic. The mucous acinus consists of mucous cells, with basal located, dark-staining, flattened nucleus. The cytoplasm stains lightly, and are vacuolated. The seromucous acinus (2) consists of both serous cells and mucous cells. In seromucous acinus, most of the cells are mucous cells, with a small amount of serous cells arranged at the end of the acinus, forming the serous semilune (3). The epithelial lining of the wall of the ducts (4) are different according to the size of the duct. In smaller ducts, simple

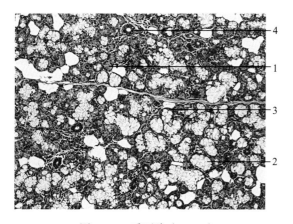

图 14-2a 舌下腺（100×）
Fig. 14-2a Sublingual gland (100×)

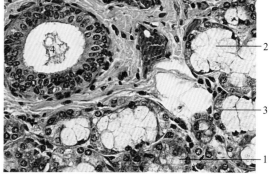

图 14-2b 舌下腺（400×）
Fig. 14-2b Sublingual gland (400×)

cuboidal or columnar epithelium can be found, while in lager ducts, tall columnar epithelium or stratified epithelium can be found.

❸ 切片 3：颌下腺

材料与方法：人颌下腺，HE 染色。

低倍镜观察：图 14-3a 显示腺实质由许多腺泡和导管（1）构成，腺泡以浆液性腺泡（2）为多，黏液性腺泡（3）和混合性腺泡（4）少。

高倍镜观察：图 14-3b 显示浆液性腺泡（1）、黏液性腺泡（2）和混合性腺泡（3）。腺泡细胞与基膜之间可见肌上皮细胞（4）。分泌管（5）发达。

3. Section 3: Submandibular gland

Materials and methods: Human submandibular gland, HE staining.

LPM: Figure 14-3a shows that the parenchyma of the gland mainly contains acini and ducts (1). Most acini are serous acini (2). There are less mucous acini (3) and seromucous acini (4).

HPM: Figure 14-3b shows serous acini (1), mucous acini (2) and seromucous acini (3). Myoepithelial cells (4) can be identified between the secretory cells and the basement membrane. The secretory ducts (5) are abundant.

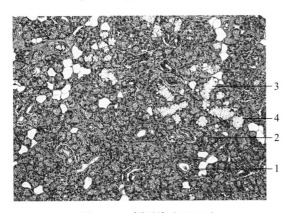 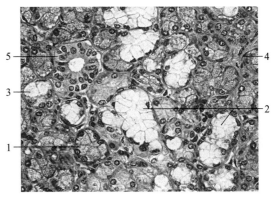

图 14-3a 颌下腺（100×）　　　　　　图 14-3b 颌下腺（400×）

Fig. 14-3a Submandibular gland (100×)　　Fig. 14-3b Submandibular gland (400×)

❹ 切片 4：胰腺

材料与方法：人或动物胰腺，HE 染色。

低倍镜观察：图 14-4a 显示腺实质被结缔组织分隔成许多大小不等的胰腺小叶。每个小叶内有许多浆液性腺泡（1）和导管（2）的断面，此为外分泌部。腺泡之间淡染的细胞团为胰岛（3）。小叶间结缔组织内可见血管（4）、淋巴管和神经节（5）。

高倍镜观察：图 14-4b 显示胰腺腺泡为纯浆液性腺泡（1），由胰腺泡细胞组成，细胞基部嗜碱性强，顶部胞质内充满细小的红色酶原颗粒。腺泡腔中可见泡心细胞（2），其胞质少，染色淡，细胞界限不清，常见一至数个浅染的细胞核。腺泡之间可找到闰管（3），细而长，管壁为单层扁平或立方上皮。胰岛（4）为球形细胞团，细胞间有丰富的毛细血管。HE 染色切片中胰岛的各种细胞不易区分。

4. Section 4: Pancreas

Materials and methods: Human or animal pancreas, HE staining.

LPM: Figure 14-4a shows that the connective tissue septae extend into the gland to divide it into lobules. The lobule is composed of exocrine and endocrine pancreas. The exocrine pancreas consists of serous acini (1) and ducts (2). The endocrine pancreas (pancreatic islet or islet of Langerhans) (3) consists of light-staining cell clusters scattered between the serous acini. Blood vessels (4), lymphatic vessels and ganglia (5) are located in the connective tissue among lobules.

HPM: Figure 14-4b shows that the pancreatic acini (1) consist of pyramidal serous cells. The basal cytoplasm is strong basophilic. In the apical cytoplasm there are many acidophilic zymogen granules. Small centroacinar cells (2) are usually found in the lumen of the acini. The centroacinar cells are flattened or cuboidal and stained pale, with light-staining nucleus. The intercalated ducts (3) are relatively long and thin, and composed of simple squamous or cuboidal epithelium. The pancreatic islets (4) are large or small clusters of endocrine cells and are stained pale. There are abundant capillaries located within the islets between the endocrine cells. In the HE-staining specimen, different kinds of endocrine cells cannot be identified.

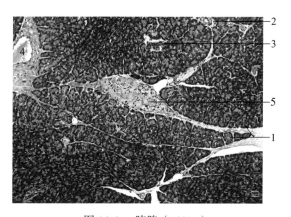

图 14-4a　胰腺（100×）
Fig. 14-4a　Pancreas (100×)

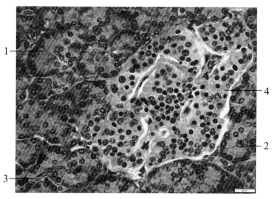

图 14-4b　胰腺（400×）
Fig. 14-4b　Pancreas (400×)

❺ 切片 5：肝

材料与方法：猪肝，HE 染色。

低倍镜观察：图 14-5a 显示多个肝小叶，肝小叶（1）呈多边形或不规则形，相邻小叶之间有较多的着色浅的结缔组织，故小叶分界明显。小叶内较大的腔隙为中央静脉（2），肝细胞在中央静脉周围呈放射状排列成肝索，肝索之间的空隙为肝血窦。相邻肝小叶之间结缔组织较多的部位为门管区（3），可见小叶间动脉、小叶间静脉和小叶间胆管的断面。

高倍镜观察：图 14-5b，肝小叶：中央静脉（1）管壁不完整。肝索（2）由 1～2 行肝细胞组成。肝细胞体积较大，为多边形；核大而圆，位于细胞中央，双核细胞较多；胞质嗜酸性，其内可见嗜碱性颗粒。肝血窦（3）形状不规则，窦壁由内皮细胞构成。有时可见内皮与肝细胞之间的窦周隙。图 14-5c，门管区：腔小壁厚的为小叶间动脉（1）；腔大壁薄，形状不规则的为小叶间静脉（2）；管壁由单层立方或柱状上皮构成的是小叶间胆管（3）。

5. Section 5: Liver

Materials and methods: Pork liver, HE staining.

LPM: Figure 14-5a shows a few hepatic lobules (1). The connective tissue invaginates from the capsule to form the septae which delineate hepatic lobules. The hepatic lobule is polygonal or irregular in shape. In the center of the lobule located the central vein (2). Plates of hepatocytes radiate outward from the central vein, forming the hepatic cords. The spaces between the hepatic cords are the hepatic sinusoids. Between hepatic lobules, connective tissue aggregates to form the portal area (3), where interlobular artery, interlobular vein, and interlobular bile duct can be seen.

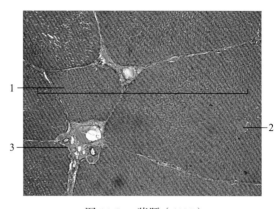

图 14-5a　猪肝（40×）
Fig. 14-5a　Pork liver (40×)

　　HPM: Figure 14-5b shows a hepatic lobule. The wall of the central vein (1) is incomplete. The hepatic cord (2) consists of 1～2 rows of hepatocytes. The hepatocyte is large and polygonal in shape, with round and large, central-located nucleus. The cytoplasm is acidophilic, with basophilic granules. Binucleated hepatocytes can be found. The hepatic sinusoid (3) has irregular lumen. It is lined by endothelial cells. Sometimes the space of Disse between sinusoidal endothelium and hepatocytes can be identified. Figure 14-5c shows the portal area. The interlobular artery (1) is the blood vessel with thick wall and small lumen. The interlobular vein (2) is the blood vessel with thin wall and large irregular lumen. The wall of the interlobular bile duct (3) is composed of simple cuboidal or columnar epithelium.

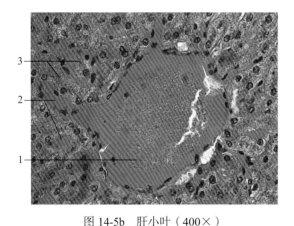

图 14-5b　肝小叶（400×）
Fig. 14-5b　Hepatic lobule (400×)

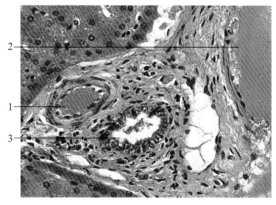

图 14-5c　门管区（400×）
Fig. 14-5c　Portal area (400×)

❻ 切片 6：肝

材料与方法：人肝，HE 染色。

低倍镜观察：图 14-6a 显示人肝和猪肝的结构基本相同，不同之处在于人肝小叶间结缔组织较少，相邻肝小叶分界不清。小叶中央的腔隙为中央静脉（1），中央静脉周围呈放射状排列的条索为肝索（2），索间间隙为肝血窦（3）。图 14-6b 显示相邻肝小叶间的结缔组织小区为门管区，可见小叶间动脉（1）、小叶间静脉（2）和小叶间胆管（3）的断面。

高倍镜观察：人肝小叶与猪肝小叶的结构基本相同。

6. Section 6: Liver

Materials and methods: Human liver, HE staining.

LPM: Figure 14-6a shows that the microscopic structures of human liver are similar to those of pig liver, except that in human liver there is less connective tissue, so that the separation between adjacent hepatic lobules is not distinctive. In the center of the hepatic lobule located the central vein (1). Plates of hepatocytes radiate outward from the central vein, forming the hepatic cords (2). The spaces between the hepatic cords are the hepatic sinusoids (3). Figure 14-6b shows that the connective tissue aggregates to form the portal area between hepatic lobules. In the portal area, interlobular artery (1), interlobular vein (2) and interlobular bile duct (3) can be seen.

HPM: The microscopic structures of human liver lobule are similar to those of pig liver lobule.

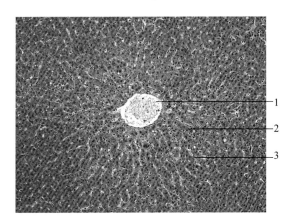

图 14-6a　人肝小叶（100×）

Fig. 14-6a　Human hepatic lobule (100×)

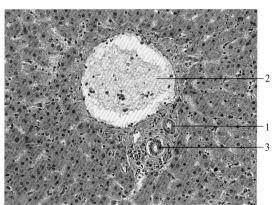

图 14-6b　人肝门管区（200×）

Fig. 14-6b　Portal area of human liver (200×)

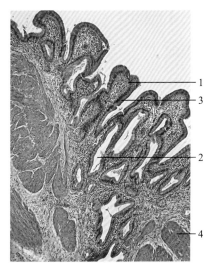

图 14-7　胆囊（100×）

Fig. 14-7　Gall bladder (100×)

❼ 切片7：胆囊

材料与方法：人胆囊，HE 染色。

低倍镜观察：图 14-7，黏膜可见许多有分支的黏膜皱襞（1），皱襞之间的上皮陷入固有层形成黏膜窦（2），有的呈封闭的腔。上皮为单层柱状（3），无杯状细胞；固有层内无腺体。肌层可见不同切面的平滑肌（4），胆囊壁没有明显的黏膜肌层，外膜为浆膜。

7. Section 7: Gall bladder

Materials and methods: Human gall bladder, HE staining.

LPM: Figure 14-7 shows that many plicae (1) can be seen in the mucosa of the gall bladder wall. Between plicae, the epithelium invaginates into the lamina propria and form sinuses (2). The epithelium is simple columnar epithelium (3) with no goblet cell. No gland exists in the lamina propria.

The muscularis propria contains interlacing bundles of smooth muscle (4). There is no distinct layer of muscularis mucosae in the gall bladder. The outside of the gall bladder is covered by serosa.

【作业】

绘制肝小叶和门管区的低倍镜结构图。

【Assignment】

Drawing to describe the structures of the hepatic lobules and the portal areas under low power microscopy.

【思考题】

1．三对唾液腺的结构与功能有何异同？
2．如何分辨腮腺和胰腺？
3．肝小叶由哪些结构组成？光镜下 HE 染色标本中哪些结构显示不清或不能显示？

【Questions】

1. What are the similarities and differences among the parotid gland, the sublingual gland, and the submandibular gland?

2. How to differentiate between the parotid gland and the pancreas?

3. What are the structures in the hepatic lobule? In HE staining section, which structures cannot be identified under light microscopy ?

【临床与科研联系英文阅读材料】 【English Reading Material for Correlations with Clinic and Scientific Research】

The development of diabetes mellitus is closely related to abnormal insulin secretion, characterized by insulin resistance and islet β-cell dysfunction. Autophagy is critical for β-cell homeostasis, particularly under conditions of stress and increased insulin demand. The stimulation of autophagy by IL-6 is regulated via multiple complementary mechanisms including inhibition of mammalian target of rapamycin complex 1 (mTORC1) and activation of Akt, ultimately leading to an increase in autophagy enzyme production. Pretreatment with IL-6 renders β cells resistant to apoptosis induced by proinflammatory cytokines, and inhibition of autophagy with chloroquine prevents the ability of IL-6 to protect from apoptosis. IL-6 can activate STAT3 and the autophagy enzyme GABARAPL1 in human islets. The direct stimulation of autophagy as a novel mechanism for IL-6-mediated protection of β cells from stress-induced apoptosis is under study.

（梁元晶　路　欣）

第15章 呼吸系统

Chapter 15 The Respiratory System

【实习内容】Contents of Observation

切片 Sections

观察切片	Observation Sections
1. 气管	1. Trachea
2. 肺	2. Lung
示教切片	Teaching Sections
3. 肺弹性纤维	3. Elastic fiber of lung
4. 气血屏障超微结构（电镜）	4. Ultrastructure of the air-blood barrier（EM）
5. Ⅱ型肺泡细胞超微结构（电镜）	5. Ultrastructure of Ⅱ-type alveolar cell（EM）

【目的要求】

1. 掌握光镜下气管和支气管的结构。
2. 掌握肺的一般结构、肺泡细胞的超微结构和功能。

【Objective】

1. To master the morphological structure of trachea and bronchi under light microscopy.
2. To master the morphological structure of lung, the ultrastructure and function of alveolar cell.

【观察切片】
【Observation Sections】

① 切片1：气管

材料与方法：猫气管，HE染色。

气管整体观察：图15-1a显示从腔面到外面，气管分为三层结构：黏膜层（1）、黏膜下层（2）和外膜层（3），外膜层含有透明软骨环（4）。软骨环缺口处为气管后壁，是气管的膜性部（5）。

1. Section 1: Trachea

Materials and methods: Trachea of cat, HE staining.

Whole mount observation of trachea: In Figure 15-1a, from the luminal surface to the outside, the trachea is divided into three layers: mucosa (1), submucosa (2) and adventitia layer (3), which contains C-shape hyaline cartilaginous ring (4). The annulus not covered by cartilage is the posterior wall of the trachea, which is the membranous portion of the trachea (5).

低倍镜观察：图15-1b显示气管的结构：①黏膜层（A），黏膜层由上皮层和固有层构成，上皮层是假复层纤毛柱状上皮（1），固有层（2）由结缔组织构成。②黏膜下层（B），黏膜下层由疏松结缔组织构成，含有大量的混合性气管腺（3）、血管等。③外膜层（C），外膜层为纤维膜，主要由透明软骨（4）和疏松结缔组织构成（5）。

LPM: Figure 15-1b shows the structure of the trachea. ① The mucosa layer (A) is composed of the epithelium and lamina propria layer. The epithelium layer is pseudostratified ciliated columnar epithelium (1). The lamina propria layer (2) is composed of connective tissue. ② The submucosal layer (B) is composed of loose connective tissue, which contains a large number of mixed tracheal glands (3), blood vessels, etc. ③ The outer layer (C) is composed of fibroelastic membrane, cartilage (4) and loose connective tissue (5).

高倍镜观察：由图15-1c可见气管黏膜层由假复层纤毛柱状上皮（1）和固有层（2）组成。上皮内含有柱状细胞（3）、梭形细胞（4）、杯状细胞（5）以及锥体细胞（6）等，柱状

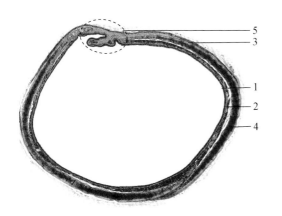

图 15-1a 气管（20×）

Fig. 15-1a Trachea (20×)

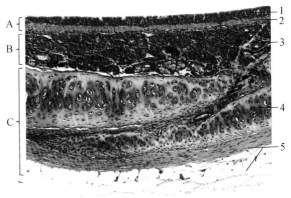

图 15-1b 气管（40×）

Fig. 15-1b Trachea (40×)

细胞游离面可见纤毛（7）。假复层纤毛柱状上皮下可见明显的基膜（8）。黏膜下层由混合腺（9）和疏松结缔组织组成，后者可见血管（10）以及脂肪等结构。

HPM: Figure 15-1c shows that the tracheal mucosa is composed of pseudostratified ciliated columnar epithelium (1) and lamina propria (2). Columnar cells (3), spindle cells (4), Goblet cells (5) and pyramidal cells (6) can be found in the epithelium, and the free cilia (7) on the columnar cells are also evident. The basement membrane (8) is evident under pseudostratified ciliated columnar epithelium. The submucosa is composed of mixed glands (9) and loose connective tissue, in which the blood vessels (10) and adipocytes can be found.

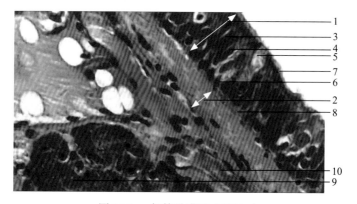

图 15-1c 气管黏膜层（400×）

Fig. 15-1c Tracheal mucosal layer (400×)

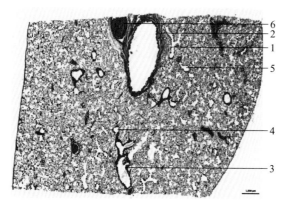

图 15-2a 肺（40×）

Fig. 15-2a Lung (40×)

❷ 切片 2：肺

材料与方法：鼠肺，HE 染色。

低倍镜观察：图 15-2a 显示肺组织切片整体观，内部大小不同的空腔为肺的各级支气管，其中比较大的腔是小支气管（1），可见散在透明软骨片（2）；依次可见细支气管（3）以及终末细支气管（4）；进一步可见呼吸性细支气管、肺泡管、肺泡囊（5）以及血管（6）。

2. Section 2: Lung

Materials and methods: Lung of mouse, HE staining.

LPM: A piece of mouse lung tissue, there are different sizes of cavities in the lung, which represent the cross-sections of bronchia, arterial and venous blood vessels (Figure 15-2a). The larger cavities are bronchia (1) and transparent cartilage (2) can be seen within the bronchial wall. Bronchioles (3) and bronchioli terminals (4) can be seen. The respiratory part including respiratory bronchioles, alveolar ducts and alveolar sacs and alveoli (5) are clearly visible. At the same time, a blood vessel (6) is near the bronchia.

高倍镜观察：肺包括导气部和呼吸部。导气部分为小支气管、细支气管以及终末细支气管。呼吸部分为呼吸性细支气管、肺泡管、肺泡囊以及肺泡。

（一）导气部

图 15-2b 显示小支气管结构，可以分为黏膜层、黏膜下层以及外膜层。

1）黏膜层：分为上皮层以及固有层。上皮层为假复层纤毛柱状上皮（1），纤毛（2）以及杯状细胞（3）明显；固有层为结缔组织。

2）黏膜下层：为疏松的结缔组织，可以看到平滑肌的断面（4）及少量腺体（5）。

3）外膜：为不连续的透明软骨（6）以及疏松的结缔组织构成。

HPM: The lung includes the conducting part and the respiratory part. The air conducting part includes small bronchia, bronchioles and bronchioli terminales. The respiratory part includes: respiratory bronchioles, alveolar ducts, alveolar sacs and alveoli.

（Ⅰ）The conducting part

Figure 15-2b is a bronchia, which can be divided into the mucosal layer, submucosal layer and the outer membrane layer.

1) Mucosal layer: Mucosa consists of epithelial layer and laminae propria. The epithelial layer is a pseudostratified ciliated columnar epithelium (1) including cilia (2) and Goblet cells (3), and laminae propria is a connective tissue layer.

2) Submucosa is composed of loose connective tissue, discrete, smooth muscle bundles (4) and a few glands (5).

3) Tunica externa layer includes discontinuous, hyaline cartilage (6) and loose connective tissue.

图 15-2c 中，（1）显示为细支气管结构。上皮层是假复层或者单层纤毛柱状上皮（2），固有层明显变薄，黏膜下层的平滑肌明显变多（3），外膜层基本看不到透明软骨。（4）显示终末细支气管，其上皮是单层纤毛柱状上皮（5），没有杯状细胞，平滑肌增多成环状，无腺体，外膜没有软骨片。

In Figure 15-2c, (1) is a bronchiole. The epithelium is pseudostratified ciliated columnar epithelium or simple ciliated columnar epithelium (2). The lamina propria is thinner and the smooth muscle of the submucosa becomes more obvious (3), the adventitial layer basically is devoid of hyaline cartilage. (4) shows bronchioles terminals, which epithelium is a single layer of columnar

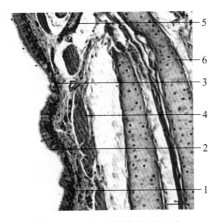

图 15-2b　小支气管（200×）

Fig. 15-2b　Small bronchia（200×）

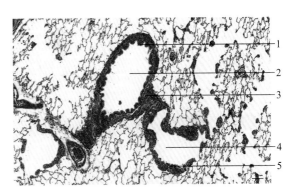

图 15-2c　细支气管和终末细支气管（100×）

Fig. 15-2c　Bronchioles and bronchioles terminals
（100×）

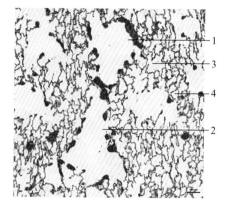

图 15-2d　肺的呼吸部（100×）

Fig. 15-2d　Respiratory portion of lung (100×)

epithelium (5), with no goblet cells. Smooth muscle increased into a ring. Glands and cartilage disappear.

（二）呼吸部

图 15-2d 显示肺的呼吸部。呼吸部是由呼吸性细支气管（1）、肺泡管（2）、肺泡囊（3）以及肺泡（4）组成。呼吸性细支气管主要由单层柱状上皮，平滑肌以及疏松结缔组织构成，外部直接连接肺泡。肺泡管由不连续的平滑肌构成，直接连接肺泡。几个肺泡连在一起构成肺泡囊。在肺泡间隔的部分常常会有吞噬了尘粒的巨噬细胞（肺里面的巨噬细胞又称尘细胞），见图 15-2e 箭头所示。肺泡间隔主要有毛细血管、少量的结缔组织；肺泡壁主要由肺的 I 型肺泡上皮细胞（图 15-2f，黄色箭头）和 II 型肺泡上皮细胞（图 15-2f，黑色箭头）组成。I 型肺泡上皮细胞呈扁平状，数量少，体积较大；II 型肺泡上皮细胞呈圆形，细胞核圆形，细胞数量多，体积较小。

（II）The respiratory part

Figure 15-2d shows the respiratory part, which is composed of respiratory bronchioles (1), alveolar ducts (2), alveolar sac (3) and alveoli (4). The respiratory bronchiole is composed of a single layer of columnar epithelium, smooth muscle and loose connective tissue. The alveolar duct is composed of discontinuous smooth muscle, which is directly connected with the alveoli. In the alveolar septum, there are usually macrophages (macrophages, also known as dust cells) in the lung (arrow of Figure 15-2e). The alveolar septum is mainly composed of capillaries and a small amount of connective tissue. The alveolar wall is mainly composed of type I alveolar epithelial cells (red arrow of Figure 15-2f) and type II alveolar epithelial cells (black arrow of Figure 15-2f). Type I alveolar epithelial cells are flat, large in size and small in quantity. type II alveolar epithelial cells are round, with round nucleus, small size and large inquantity.

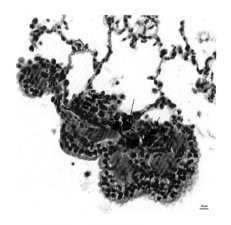

图 15-2e　肺巨噬细胞（200×）

Fig. 15-2e　Pulmonary macrophages (200×)

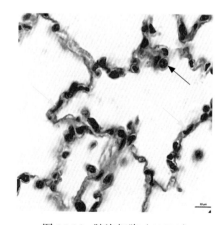

图 15-2f　肺泡细胞（400×）

Fig. 15-2f　Alveolar epithelial cells (400×)

【示教切片】
【Teaching Sections】

❸ 切片 3：肺弹性纤维

材料与方法：猫肺组织，地衣红染色。

弹性纤维含量较胶原纤维少，但分布较广。图 15-3 中，在肺组织中弹性纤维经地衣红染色，呈棕红色或深棕色。

3. Section 3: Elastic fiber of lung

Materials and methods: Lung of cat orcein staining.

Elastic fiber content is less than collagen fiber, but the distribution is wide. In Figure 15-3, Elastic fibers of the lung tissue are brown-red or dark brown with Orcein staining.

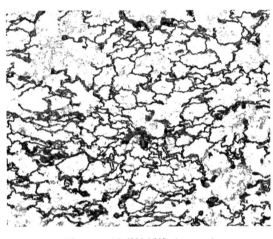

图 15-3　肺弹性纤维（100×）
Fig. 15-3　Lung elastic fibers (100×)

❹ 切片 4：气血屏障

材料与方法：鼠肺，用锇酸固定制片。

图 15-4 显示了电子显微镜下气血屏障的主要三层结构。这三层结构分别是毛细血管内皮细胞层（1）；基底膜（两个细胞共用一个融合的基底膜）（2），肺泡与肺部毛细血管紧密相连，两者的膜大部分融合，有助于气体的快速扩散；肺泡上皮细胞层（3）。

4. Section 4: Blood-air barrier

Materials and methods: Lung of mouse, slices made of osmium acid.

This electron micrograph of Figure 15-4 shows the three layers of the air-blood barrier. It consists of three layers: the endothelial cell represents the capillary epithelium (1); alveolar epithelial cell and endothelial cell layer share a fused basement membrane (2), which allows for the minimization of the barrier across which exchange must occur; and the type I pneumocyte (3).

❺ 切片 5：肺泡细胞超微结构（电镜）

图 15-5 显示肺泡 II 型上皮细胞。电镜下，II 型肺泡细胞的细胞核明显（1），细胞游离面有少量的微绒毛（2），胞质内富含线粒体和溶酶体，有较发达的粗面内质网和高尔基复合体。核上方有嗜锇性板层小体（3）。

5. Section 5: The ultrastructure of alveolar cells pneumocytes (electron micrograph)

Figure 15-5 shows type II pneumocytes. They are obvious nucleus (1), the free surfaces of the cells have a small amount of microvilli (2) under electron microscopy. Mitochondria, lysosomes, rough endoplasmic reticulum and Golgi complex are rich in their cytoplasm. Above the nucleus, there are osmilphilic multilamellar bodies (3).

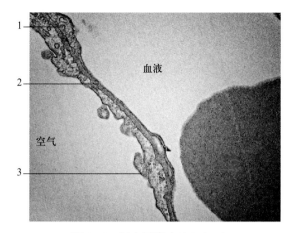

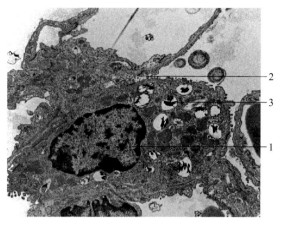

图 15-4　气血屏障（40 000×）
Fig. 15-4　Blood-air barrier (40 000×)

图 15-5　Ⅱ型肺泡细胞（12 000×）
Fig. 15-5　Type Ⅱ alveolar cells (12 000×)

【作业】

绘制肺呼吸部结构。

【Assignment】

To draw the histological structure of pulmonary respiration part.

【思考题】

1．试述肺泡隔的超微结构及其与呼吸功能的关系。
2．试述呼吸系统净化空气和防御功能有关的结构。

【Questions】

1. To describe the ultrastructure of alveolar septa and its role in respiratory function.
2. To describe the structure involved in cleaning air and defending in respiratory system.

【临床与科研联系英文阅读材料】
【English Reading Material for Correlations with Clinic and Scientific Research】

The smooth muscle layer of bronchioles is controlled by the parasympathetic nervous system. Normally, the smooth muscle coats contract at the end of expiration and relax during inspiration. In persons with asthma, however, the smooth muscle coat undergoes prolonged contraction during expiration; thus, these individuals have difficulty in inhaling air into their lungs. Steroids and β_2-agonists relax bronchiolar smooth muscle and are frequently used to relieve asthmatic attacks.

（任芳丽　王大亮）

第16章 泌尿系统

Chapter 16 Urinary System

【实习内容】Contents of Observation

切片　Sections

观察切片	Observation Sections
1. 肾脏	1. Kidney
2. 膀胱	2. Urinary bladder
3. 输尿管	3. Ureter

【目的要求】

1. 掌握肾的结构特点，在光镜下正确辨认。
2. 掌握膀胱和输尿管的结构特点，在光镜下正确辨认。

【Objective】

1. To master morphological characteristics of the kidney, and correctly identify them under light microscopy.

2. To master morphological features of urinary bladder and ureter, and correctly identify them under light microscopy.

【观察切片】
【Observation Sections】

1 切片 1：肾脏

材料与方法：人肾脏，HE 染色。

低倍镜观察：图 16-1a，肾实质分皮质和髓质。皮质染色较深，可见皮质迷路（1）和髓放线（2）；髓质（3）内有密集排列的小管。

高倍镜观察：图 16-1b，肾皮质内的圆形结构为肾小体，血管球（1）位于肾小体中，为成团的毛细血管。肾小体外周的单层扁平上皮为肾小囊壁层，肾小囊脏层为足细胞，因与毛细血管内皮紧密相贴不易分清。肾小囊脏、壁层之间较窄的腔为肾小囊腔（2）。肾小体周围有许多近端小管曲部（3）和远端小管曲部（4）的各种断面。近端小管曲部管腔小而不规则，上皮细胞为锥体形，细胞界限不清，核圆形位于细胞基部，胞质嗜酸性强染成红色。细胞游离面可见整齐的刷状缘。远端小管曲部管腔大而规则，管壁薄由单层立方上皮构成，染色浅，细胞界限清楚，核圆形位于细胞中央。可见远端小管靠近肾小体侧的上皮细胞呈柱状，排列紧密，为致密斑（5）。

图 16-1c，肾髓质主要由肾小管和集合小管组成，其中含少量结缔组织及血管。可见近端小管直部（1）与远端小管直部（2），结构分别与其曲部相似。细段（3）：管腔小，管壁由单层扁平上皮构成，细胞含核部分较厚。集合小管（4）：管腔大，管壁由单层立方或柱状上皮构成，细胞界限清楚，染色较淡。

1. Section 1: Kidney

Materials and methods: Human kidney, HE staining.

LPM: In Figure 16-1a the renal parenchyma is divided into cortex and medulla. The cortex is dark staining. Cortical labyrinths (1) and medullary rays (2) can be seen. The medulla (3) consists of tubules and ducts.

HPM: In Figure 16-1b many round renal corpuscles can be found in the cortex. In the renal corpuscle, glomeruli are present (1) as a tuft of capillaries. The outermost part of the renal corpuscle is simple flattened squamous epithelium, which is referred as the parietal layer of Bowman's capsule. The visceral layer of Bowman's capsule is composed of podocytes, which are not easy to be identified in HE staining sections. Between the parietal and visceral layers is a narrow space, the lumen of Bowman's capsule (2). Adjacent to the renal corpuscles are proximal convoluted tubules (3) and distal convoluted tubules (4). The lumen of the proximal convoluted tubule is small and irregular. The wall of the tubule is composed of a layer of pyramidal cells with acidophilic cytoplasm and basally located round nuclei. The lateral boundaries of the cells are not clear. Brush border can be found on the free surface of the cells. The lumen of the distal convoluted tubule is large and regular. The wall of the tubule is thicker, regularer and composed of a layer of cuboidal cells with distinct cell boundaries, light-staining cytoplasm, and round, centrally located nuclei The macula densa (5) is an area of closely packed, specialized cells lining the distal convoluted tubule where it abuts the glomerular vascular pole.

Figure 16-1c, the renal medulla is mainly composed of renal tubules and collecting tubules. Between the tubules are small amount of connective tissue and blood vessels. Proximal straight tubules (1) and distal straight tubules (2) are seen. The structure of proximal straight tubule is similar to that of proximal convoluted tubule, while the structure of distal straight tubule is similar to that of distal convoluted tubule. Thin segment (3) has a very small lumen and a thin wall composed of simple flattened epithelium. Collecting tubule (4) has a big lumen. The wall

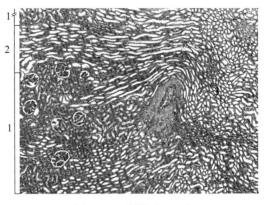

图 16-1a   肾脏（40×）

Fig. 16-1a   Kidney (40×)

consists of simple cuboidal or columnar epithelium, with clear cell boundaries and light-staining cytoplasm.

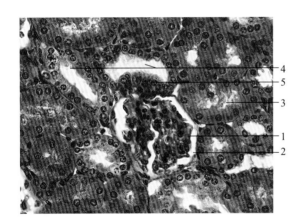

图 16-1b   肾皮质（400×）

Fig. 16-1b   Renal cortex (400×)

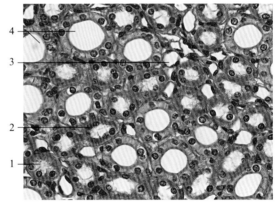

图 16-1c   肾髓质（400×）

Fig. 16-1c   Renal medulla (400×)

❷ 切片 2：膀胱

材料与方法：动物膀胱，HE 染色。

低倍镜观察：图 16-2，膀胱壁由内向外分黏膜（1）、肌层（2）和外膜（3）。黏膜由上皮（4）和固有层（5）构成。上皮为变移上皮。固有层位于变移上皮下方，由结缔组织构成。肌层由内纵、中环、外纵平滑肌构成。外膜大部分为纤维膜，顶部为浆膜。

2. Section 2: Urinary bladder

Materials and methods: Animal urinary bladder, HE staining.

LPM: In Figure 16-2, the wall of urinary bladder consists of mucosa (1), muscularis (2) and adventitia (3). Mucosa is composed of epithelium (4) and lamina propria (5). The epithelium of the urinary bladder is transitional epithelium. The lamina propria is located underneath the trunsitional epithelium, containing connective tissue. The muscularis consists of 3 layers of smooth muscle, inner and outer longitudinal and middle circular layers. The adventitia is composed of connective tissue or apical serosa.

❸ 切片 3：输尿管

材料与方法：动物输尿管，HE 染色。

低倍镜观察：图 16-3，输尿管管壁由内向外分黏膜（1）、肌层（2）及外膜（3）。各层结构与膀胱类似，但肌层较薄，由内环、外纵两层平滑肌构成。

3. Section 3: Ureter

Materials and methods: Animal ureter, HE staining.

LPM: In Figure 16-3 inside-out the wall of ureter consists of mucosa (1), muscularis (2) and adventitia (3), which are similar to those of urinary bladder, except that the muscularis is thinner, containing only 2 layers of smooth muscle, inner circular and outer longitudinal layers.

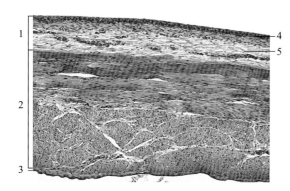

图 16-2　膀胱（100×）

Fig. 16-2　Urinary bladder (100×)

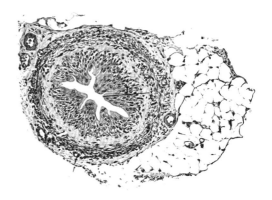

图 16-3　输尿管（100×）

Fig. 16-3　Ureter (100×)

【作业】

绘图描述肾皮质高倍镜结构。

【Assignment】

Drawing to describe morphological structures of kidney cortex under high power microscopy.

【思考题】

1．试述肾皮质和髓质的结构特点。
2．试述膀胱壁的结构特点。
3．试述输尿管管壁的结构特点。

【Questions】

1. To describe structural features of cortex and medulla of the kidney.

2. To describe structural features of the wall of the urinary bladder.

3. To describe structural features of the wall of the ureter.

【临床与科研联系英文阅读材料】
【English Reading Material for Correlations with Clinic and Scientific Research】

The kidney is an essential mammalian organ that serves to filter toxins and metabolic by-products out of the blood, which are then excreted through urine. Hydrogen sulphide (H_2S) is a recently characterized, endogenous gaseous molecule with important physiological roles. Many interesting roles continue to be revealed for H_2S related specifically to the kidney. H_2S plays a complex and essential role in the normal function of the kidney and dysregulation of H_2S production can directly or indirectly contribute to the pathogenesis of renal disease and injury. Also, H_2S could be a promising potential therapeutic treatment to reduce the severity of several renal diseases.

（梁元晶　路　欣）

第17章 男性生殖系统

Chapter 17 Male Reproductive System

【实习内容】Contents of Observation

 切片 Sections

观察切片	Observation Sections
1. 睾丸及附睾	1. Testis and epididymis
2. 输精管	2. Deferens
3. 前列腺	3. Prostate
示教切片	Teaching Sections
4. 精囊	4. Seminal vesicle

【目的要求】

1. 掌握睾丸的结构及精子发生过程中生精细胞的结构变化。
2. 掌握附睾的结构。
3. 掌握输精管的结构。
4. 掌握前列腺的结构。
5. 掌握精子的结构。
6. 了解精囊的结构特点。

【Objective】

1. To master the structure of testis and the changes of the spermatogenic cells in the process of

spermatogenesis.

2. To master the structure of epididymis.

3. To master the structure of deferens.

4. To master the structure of prostate.

5. To master the structure of sperm.

6. To understand the structural characteristics of seminal vesicle.

【观察切片】
【Observation Sections】

❶ 切片 1：睾丸和附睾

材料与方法：人睾丸和附睾，HE 染色。

（1）睾丸

1）睾丸被膜

高倍镜观察：图 17-1a 显示睾丸被膜。睾丸被膜由鞘膜脏层（1），白膜（2）和血管膜（与睾丸间质相连）组成，有时鞘膜腔（3）可见。

1. Section 1: Testis and epididymis

Materials and methods: Human testis and epididymis, HE staining.

(1) Testis

1) Capsule of testis

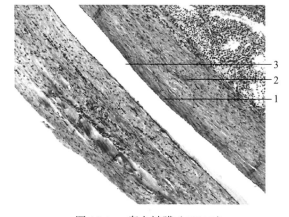

图 17-1a　睾丸被膜（400×）
Fig. 17-1a　Capsule of testis (400×)

HPM: Figure 17-1a shows capsule of testis. The capsule of testis contains perididymis (1), tunica albuginea (2) and laminae vasculosa testis . Sometimes it is visible for the cavity of tunica vaginalis (3).

2）睾丸实质

低和高倍镜观察：图 17-1b 显示睾丸实质主要由生精小管（1）组成，生精小管之间的结缔组织为睾丸间质。图 17-1c 显示生精小管基部为一层染为粉红色的基膜（1），管壁由复层生精上皮组成（2）。生精小管内部为管腔（3），生精小管之间为间质（4）。图 17-1d 显示睾丸白膜在与附睾相接部位增厚为睾丸纵隔（1），纵隔内的网状裂隙即睾丸网（2），图中（3）显示生精小管。图 17-1e 显示生精小管（1）在近睾丸纵隔处变为直精小管（2），图中（3）显示血管。

2) Parenchyma of testis

LPM / HPM: Figure 17-1b shows testis, which mainly contains seminiferous tubules (1). The connective tissue between spermatogenic tubules is testicular interstitial tissue. Figure 17-1c shows basement membrane (1) and the seminiferous epithelium (2). The inner part of the spermatogenic tubule is the lumen (3), and the outer part is the interstitium (4). Figure 17-1d Rete testis forms a sponge-like network in the mediastinum. The junction between tunica albuginea of testis and the epididymis was thickened to the mediastinum of the testis (1). The reticular fissure in the

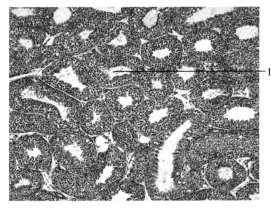

图 17-1b　睾丸（40×）

Fig. 17-1b　Testis (40×)

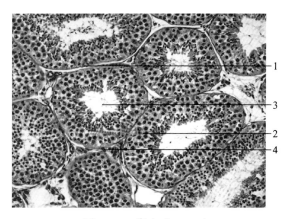

图 17-1c　睾丸（100×）

Fig. 17-1c　Testis (100×)

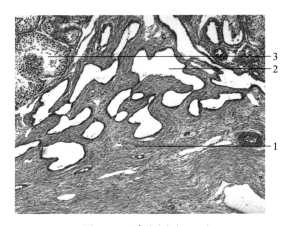

图 17-1d　睾丸网（40×）

Fig. 17-1d　Rete testis（40×）

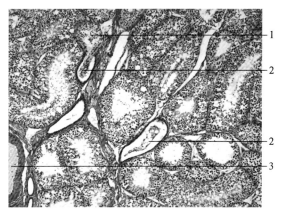

图 17-1e　直精小管（400×）

Fig. 17-1e　Tubulus rectus (400×)

mediastinum is the reticulum testis (2), (3) shows seminiferous tubule . Figure 17-1e shows that the sperm tube (1) becomes a straight tube (2). (3) shows the blood vessel.

　　3）生精小管

　　高倍镜：观察生精小管中各级生精细胞和支持细胞等的形态结构特点。图 17-1f、图 17-1g、图 17-1h 显示生精上皮中处于不同发育阶段的各级生精细胞、支持细胞及肌样细胞等。精原细胞（1），紧贴基膜，呈圆形或椭圆形，体积较小。初级精母细胞（2），体积大，呈圆形，细胞核大，染色质呈丝球状。次级精母细胞，细胞体积较小，呈圆形，细胞核染色较深，也呈圆形。因迅速进入第二次减数分裂，存在时间较短，在切片中不多见。精子细胞（3）（圆形精子细胞），靠近管腔，体积小，细胞核圆而小，染色较深。精子（4），处于变态期的各级精子，主要可见变长深染的头部（包括长形精子细胞）。支持细胞（5），轮廓不清，细胞质染色浅，细胞核形态不规则，染色质着色浅，核仁明显。肌样细胞（6），紧贴基膜的梭形细胞。

　　3) Seminiferous tubules

　　HPM: Figures 17-1f, 17-1g and 17-1h show the spermatogenic cells at different developmental stage, sertoli cells, and myoid cells. Spermatogonia (1) are at the tubule base, and they are relatively small cells with a relatively large spherical nucleus. Primary spermatocytes (2) are the largest cells of spermatogenic lineage and characterized by the presence of chromosomes in different stages of the coiling process within their nuclei. Secondary spermatocytes are difficult to observe in sections because they remain very briefly and enter quickly into the second meiotic division. They are relatively small round cells with darkly stained nuclei. Round Spermatid (3) can be distinguished by their small size, nuclei with areas of condensed chromatin, and juxta-luminal location within the tubules. Spermatozoon (4) (elongated spermatids) are elongated cells with darkly stained head. Sertoli cells (5) are irregularly columnar cells, with borders that are hard to distinguish, and they have jagged, euchromatic nucleus with a prominent nucleolus. Myoid cells (6) are surrounded with a thin outer capsule.

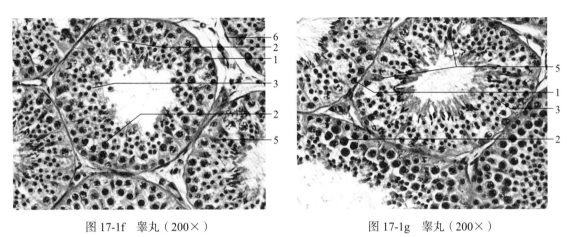

图 17-1f 睾丸（200×）   图 17-1g 睾丸（200×）
Fig. 17-1f   Testis (200×)   Fig. 17-1g   Testis (200×)

4）间质细胞

高倍镜观察：图 17-1i 和图 17-1j 所示为睾丸间质细胞（箭头所示）。位于生精小管之间的结缔组织内，常成群存在。细胞体积较大，胞质嗜酸性，细胞核圆形，常偏位，染色浅，核仁明显。

4) Leydig cells of testis

HPM: Figure 17-1i and 17-1j show Leydig cells of testis (arrows). Clusters of Leydig cells

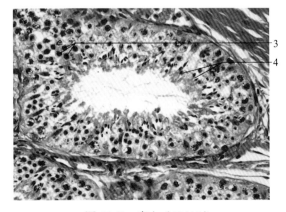

图 17-1h 睾丸（200×）
Fig. 17-1h   Testis (200×)

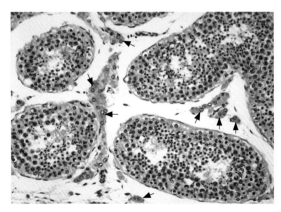

图 17-1i 间质细胞（箭头所指，100×）
Fig. 17-1i   Leydig cells (arrows, 100×)

(interstitial cells) occupy angular spaces in the stroma. They are lightly eosinophilic and have a foamy cytoplasm, eccentric spherical nuclei with prominent nucleoli.

5）直精小管

高倍镜观察：图 17-1k 显示生精小管（1）和直精小管（2）相连处，可见复层生精上皮变为单层柱状或立方上皮。

5) Tubulus Rectus

HPM: Figure 17-1k shows the junction of seminiferous tubules (1) and tubulus rectus (2), where seminiferous epithelium becomes simple columnar or cuboidal epithelium.

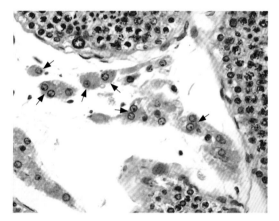

图 17-1j　间质细胞（箭头所指，200×）

Fig. 17-1j　Leydig cells (arrows, 200×)

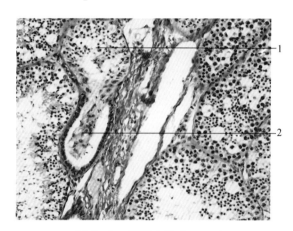

图 17-1k　直精小管（100×）

Fig. 17-1k　Tubulus rectus (100×)

（2）附睾

低倍镜观察：图 17-1l 显示附睾输出小管（1）断面，位于附睾头部。管腔起伏不平，管壁被覆纤毛柱状上皮。图 17-1m 显示附睾管断面，位于附睾体部和尾部。管腔平整，管壁被覆假复层柱状上皮（1），管腔内有精子（2）。

(2) Epididymis

LPM: Figure 17-1l shows efferent ducts (1) that are in the head of epididymis, lined by ciliated columnar epithelium. Figure 17-1m shows epididymal ducts that are in the body and tail of

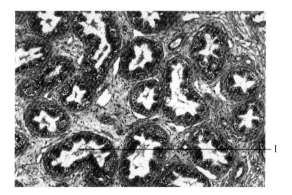

图 17-1l　输出小管（40×）

Fig. 17-1l　Efferent ducts (40×)

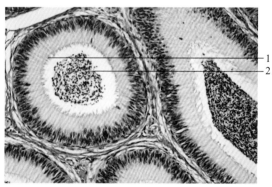

图 17-1m　附睾管（100×）

Fig. 17-1m　Epididymal ducts (100×)

epididymis, which consist of tall pseudostratified epithelium (1). There are sperms (2) in the lumen.

高倍镜观察：图 17-1n 显示输出小管上皮中的低柱状无纤毛细胞（1）和高柱状纤毛细胞（2）；两种细胞交错排列，使输出小管腔面起伏不平。图 17-1o 显示附睾管上皮细胞表面有整齐排列的静纤毛（1）；柱状细胞（2）呈高柱状，细胞核椭圆，色浅；基细胞（3）位于基膜上。管腔中储存大量精子（4）。

HPM: Figure 17-1n shows that epithelium of efferent duct consists of low columnar cell without stereocilia (1) and high columnar cell with stereocilia (2). Figure 17-1o shows that the epithelial cells of the epididymis are lined with neatly arranged stereocilia (1). The lining cells (2) are tall columnar with elliptic nuclei. Basal cells (3) are located on basement membrane. Large number of sperms (4) are in the lumen.

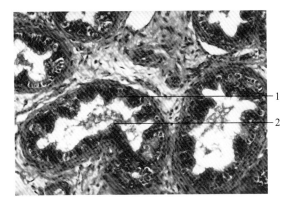

图 17-1n　输出小管（100×）

Fig. 17-1n　Efferent ducts (100×)

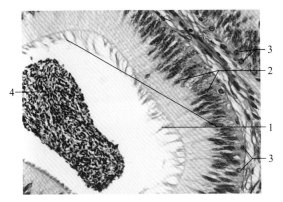

图 17-1o　附睾管（200×）

Fig. 17-1o　Epididymal ducts (200×)

② 切片 2：输精管

材料与方法：人输精管，HE 染色。

低倍镜观察：图 17-2a 显示输精管的横断面，从内向外由黏膜（1）、肌层（2）和外膜三层组成。肌层较厚，由内纵、中环、外纵三层平滑肌组成。外膜为结缔组织。

高倍镜观察：图 17-2b 显示输精管黏膜为假复层柱状上皮（1），与附睾管相似，有静纤毛（2）。

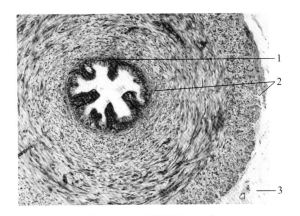

图 17-2a　输精管（40×）

Fig. 17-2a　Ductus deferens (40×)

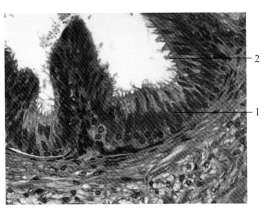

图 17-2b　输精管（200×）

Fig. 17-2b　Ductus deferens (200×)

2. Section 2: Deferens

Materials and methods: Human deferens, HE staining.

LPM: Figure 17-2a is the transverse section of the ductus deferens, which consists of three layers: mucosa (1), three-layer smooth muscle (2) and adventitia of connective tissue.

HPM: Figure 17-2b shows that the mucosa of ductus deferens consists of pseudostratified columnar epithelium (1), similar to epididymis, with static cilia (2).

❸ 切片 3：前列腺

材料与方法：人前列腺，HE 染色。

低倍镜观察：图 17-3a 显示前列腺的腺泡形态不规则，皱襞较多。腺泡腔内可见红染的前列腺凝固体（箭头所示）。腺泡之间由结缔组织和平滑肌组成。

高倍镜观察：图 17-3b 显示前列腺腺泡上皮形态多样，可以是单层立方、单层柱状或假复层柱状上皮。

3. Section 3: Prostate

Materials and methods: Human prostate, HE staining.

LPM: Figure 17-3a shows that the lining glandular epithelium is irregularly folded. Prostatic concretions (arrow) can be seen in the alveolar lumen. Underlying stroma is a mixture of smooth muscle and connective tissue.

HPM: Figure 17-3b shows that the glandular epithelium of the prostate might be pseudostratified epithelium, simple cuboidal or columnar epithelium.

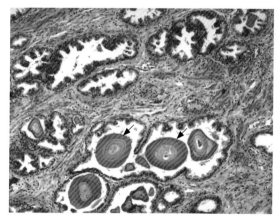 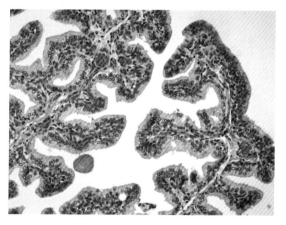

图 17-3a　前列腺（40×）　　　　　　图 17-3b　前列腺（100×）
Fig. 17-3a　Prostate (40×)　　　　　Fig. 17-3b　Prostate (100×)

【示教切片】
【Teaching Sections】

❹ 切片 4：精囊

材料与方法：人精囊，HE 染色。

低倍镜观察：图 17-4a 显示精囊黏膜向腔内凸起形成高大的皱襞，皱襞彼此融合，将囊腔分为许多彼此通连的小腔。

高倍镜观察：图 17-4b 显示精囊黏膜表面为单层柱状或假复层柱状上皮。

4. Section 4: Seminal vesicle

Materials and methods: Human seminal vesicle, HE staining.

LPM: Figure 17-4a shows that the seminal vesicle is irregularly shaped with the epithelium forming high folds.

HPM: Figure 17-4b shows that the glandular epithelium of the seminal vesicles is pseudostratified or simple columnar epithelium.

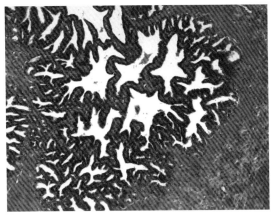

图 17-4a　精囊（40×）

Fig. 17-4a　Seminal vesicles (40×)

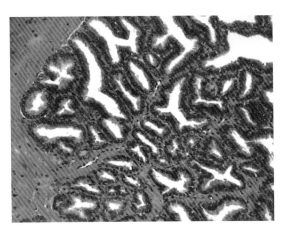

图 17-4b　精囊（100×）

Fig. 17-4b　Seminal vesicles (100×)

【作业】

绘图并描述支持细胞的组织结构。

【Assignment】

To draw and describe the histological structure of sertoli cells.

【思考题】

1. 什么是精子形成？
2. 试述睾丸间质细胞组织结构特点及功能。
3. 试述精子的光镜及电镜结构。

【Questions】

1. What is the spermatogenesis?

2. Try to describe the histological features and function of leydig cells.

3. Try to describe the structure of spermatozoa.

【临床与科研联系英文阅读材料】
【English Reading Material for Correlations with Clinic and Scientific Research】

Benign prostatic hypertrophy is a common clinical condition affecting many men older than 50 years. It is caused by hyperplasia of glandular and stromal cells in the prostate and leads to non-malignant enlargement of the gland. Periurethral nodules may compress the urethra so that urine flow is reduced and the bladder is difficult to empty. The frequency and severity of benign prostatic hypertrophy increase with aging.

（徐　健）

第 18 章 女性生殖系统

Chapter 18 Female Reproductive System

【实习内容】Contents of Observation

切片 Sections

观察切片	Observation Sections
1. 卵巢	1. Ovary
2. 输卵管	2. fallopian tube
3. 子宫及子宫内膜（增生期）	3. Uterus & endometrium（proliferative phase）
4. 子宫内膜（分泌期）	4. Endometrium（secretory phase）
5. 子宫颈	5. Cervix
6. 乳腺（静止期）	6. Mammary gland（stationary phase）
7. 乳腺（分泌期）	7. Mammary gland（secretory phase）
示教切片	**Teaching Sections**
8. 妊娠黄体	8. Corpora luteum of pregnancy

【目的要求】

1. 掌握卵巢的结构及卵泡发育过程的结构变化。
2. 了解输卵管的结构与功能，输卵管黏膜上皮细胞的类型。
3. 掌握子宫的结构；比较增生期与分泌期子宫内膜的光镜结构特点。
4. 掌握子宫颈的光镜结构特点。
5. 熟悉静止期与分泌期乳腺的不同结构特点。

【 Objective 】

1. To master the morphological characteristics of ovary and the histological changes during the development of ovarian follicles.

2. To understand the morphology and function of fallopian tube, and to know the cell types of mucosal epithelium of fallopian tube.

3. To master the uterine morphology, and compare the morphological differences of endometrium between proliferative phase and secretory phase under LM.

4. To master the morphological features of cervix under LM.

5. To be familiar with the morphological features of mammary glands on resting and secretory phases.

【观察切片】
【 Observation Sections 】

① 切片 1：卵巢

材料与方法：猫卵巢，HE 染色。

低倍镜观察：图 18-1a 显示卵巢整体的组织结构，显示卵巢由皮质（A）和髓质（B）组成。卵巢表面覆盖有被膜（1），皮质中含有各级卵泡（2）、黄体（3）以及白体等。髓质由含有卵巢血管（4）、神经和淋巴管分支的结缔组织组成。

1. Section 1: Ovary

Material and Methods: Ovary of the cat, HE staining.

LPM: Figure 18-1a shows the gross view of the ovary, which consists of the cortex (A) and medulla (B). The surface of the ovary is covered by serous membrane (1). The cortex contains follicles (2) at different development phases, the corpora lutea (3) and the corpora albicans. The medulla consists of connective tissue containing branches of ovarian blood vessels (4), nerves, and lymphatics.

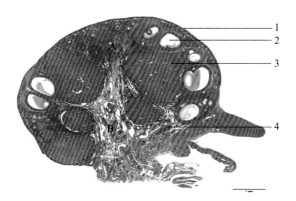

图 18-1a　卵巢（10×）
Fig. 18-1a　Ovary（10×）

高倍镜观察：观察各个阶段卵泡的镜下结构特点。

（1）原始卵泡：图 18-1b 显示原始卵泡（↗）存在于富有细胞密集的结缔组织基质（CT）中。初级卵母细胞（1）的细胞核（2）大，偏于一侧，核仁明显。可观察到初级卵母细胞的细胞质（3）和外层的扁平卵泡细胞（4）。

HPM: To observe the microscopic structural characteristics of follicles in different stages.

(1) Primordial Follicles: Figure 18-1b shows primordial follicles (↗) existed in a richly cellular connective tissue stroma (CT). The primary oocyte (1) has a large, eccentric nucleus (2) with distinct nucleolus and rich cytoplasm (3). There is a single layer of flatten follicular cells (4) surrounding the primary oocyte.

（2）初级卵泡：图 18-1c 显示初级卵泡由初级卵母细胞（1）及外层单层或多层卵泡细胞（2）组成。透明带（3），原始卵泡（4）及基质（5）可见。

(2) Primary Follicle: Figure 18-1c shows a primary follicle, which consists of primary oocyte (1) and the multi-layered granulosa cells (2). Zona pellucida (3), primordial follicles (4) and stroma (5) also can be observed.

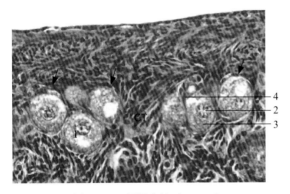 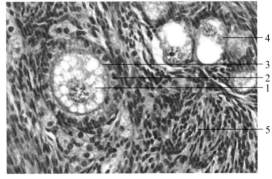

图 18-1b　原始卵泡（400×）　　　　　图 18-1c　初级卵泡（400×）

Fig. 18-1b　Primordial follicle (400×)　　　Fig. 18-1c　Primary follicle (400×)

（3）次级卵泡：图 18-1d 显示次级卵泡。初级卵母细胞（1）的细胞质呈弱嗜酸性，其周围是透明带（2）。多层的卵泡细胞间出现充满液体的卵泡腔（3），将卵泡细胞分为两部分，初级卵母细胞周围的细胞称作放射冠（4），而卵泡腔周边的细胞称作颗粒层（5）。基膜（6）将颗粒细胞与卵泡膜分隔开来。卵泡膜由卵泡周围的结缔组织细胞逐渐分化而成。

(3) Secondary Follicle: Figure 18-1d shows a secondary follicle. The oocyte has (1) a pale, eosinophilic cytoplasm, surrounded by the zona pellucida (2). A liquid-filled antrum (3) can be observed between multiple layers of follicular cells. The follicular cells are divided into two parts, the cells surrounding the primary oocyte are called radial corona (4), and the cells surrounding the follicular cavity are called granular layer (5). A basal lamina (6) separates the multi-layered mass of granulosa cells from the theca. The follicular theca is formed by the gradual differentiation of connective tissue cells around the follicle.

（4）成熟卵泡（格拉夫卵泡）：图 18-1e 显示一格拉夫卵泡。可见卵泡腔（1）增大，初级卵母细胞（2）及放射冠（3）被挤到卵泡的一端，卵丘结构明显。颗粒层（4）变薄，卵泡膜（5）发育充分。

(4) Mature follicle (Graafian follicle): Figure 18-1e shows a Graafian follicle. The follicular cavity (1) is enlarged, the primary oocyte (2) and the corona radiata (3) are squeezed into one end of the follicle, and the cumulus oophorus is prominent. The granular layer (4) becomes thinner and the follicular theca (5) is fully developed.

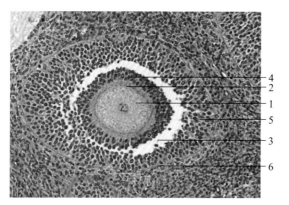

图 18-1d　次级卵泡（200×）

Fig. 18-1d　Secondary follicle（200×）

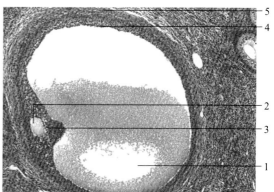

图 18-1e　格拉夫卵泡（100×）

Fig. 18-1e　Graafian follicle（100×）

（5）闭锁卵泡：图 18-1f 显示次级卵泡阶段的两个闭锁卵泡（1）。可见初级卵母细胞（2）发生萎缩，颗粒细胞分散（3），细胞核固缩，其外为着色浅、体积较大的卵泡膜细胞（4）包绕。

(5) Atretic follicle: Figure 18-1f shows atretic follicles (1), which consist of atrophic oocytes (2) and disaggregated granulosa cells (3), surrounding by pale and large sized theca cells (4).

（6）间质腺：图 18-1g 显示一间质腺（1）。生长卵泡退化后，周围肥大的卵泡膜内层细胞（2）成团地分散在结缔组织中。

(6) Interstitial gland: Figure 18-1g shows an interstitial gland (1). After the regression of follicle, the periphery corpulent theca interna cells (2) disperse in clumps in connective tissue.

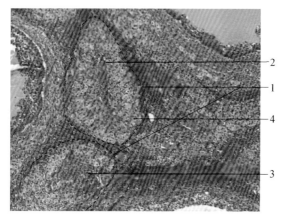

图 18-1f　闭锁卵泡（100×）

Fig. 18-1f　Atretic follicle (100×)

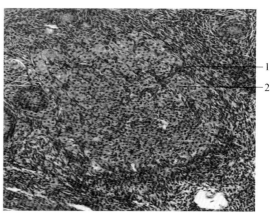

图 18-1g　间质腺（100×）

Fig. 18-1g　Interstitial gland (100×)

（7）黄体：图18-1h显示一黄体（1），主要由颗粒黄体细胞组成（2）；图18-1i显示高倍镜下黄体含有颗粒黄体细胞和膜黄体细胞两种类型。其中颗粒黄体细胞（▲）的细胞核呈圆形，胞质弱嗜酸性，略淡染。膜黄体细胞（✎）体积略小，染色较深，多位于结缔组织与血管之间。

(7) Corpus luteum: Figure 18-1h shows a corpus (1), which mainly consists of granulosa lutein cells (2). Figure 18-1i shows a corpus luteum containing granulosa lutein cells and theca lutein cells. The granulosa lutein cells (▲) have round nuclei and pale eosinophilic

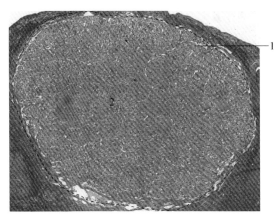

图 18-1h　黄体（100×）

Fig. 18-1h　Corpus luteum (100×)

cytoplasm. The theca lutein cells (✎) are smaller than the granulosa lutein cells with deeper staining and are located close to the connective tissue and blood vessels.

（8）白体：图18-1j显示白体（1）为结缔组织瘢痕。

(8) Corpus albicans: Figure 18-1j shows a corpus albicans (1) which appears as an involuted connective tissue scar.

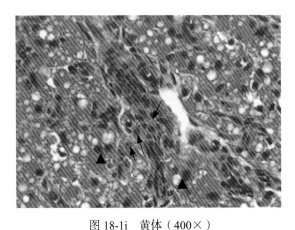

图 18-1i　黄体（400×）

Fig. 18-1i　Corpus luteum (400×)

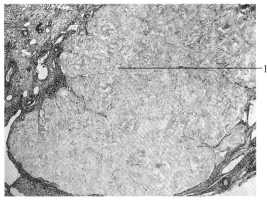

图 18-1j　白体（100×）

Fig. 18-1j　Corpus albicans (100×)

❷ 切片2：输卵管

材料与方法：人输卵管，HE染色。

低倍镜观察：图18-2a显示输卵管的横切面呈管腔样结构。从内向外依次为黏膜层，分为黏膜上皮层（1）和由结缔组成构成的固有层（2）；并向管腔（3）内突出形成黏膜皱襞（4）；肌层（5），由内环外纵的平滑肌组成；浆膜层（6）。

2. Section 2: Fallopian tube

Materials and methods: Fallopian tube of human, paraffin embedding, HE staining.

LPM: Figure 18-2a shows a fallopian tube at the level of the ampulla in transverse section. The wall of a fallopian tube from inner to outer are: mucosa, consisting of an epithelium (1) and a lamina propria (2), which protrudes into the lumen (3) and forms the mucosa folds (4) ; muscularis (5), consisting of two layers of smooth muscle-an inner circular and an outer longitudinal; and serosa (6).

高倍镜观察：图 18-2b 显示输卵管的柱状上皮主要由两种细胞组成：纤毛细胞（1），细胞表面有纤毛朝向子宫方向摆动；分泌细胞（2），无纤毛。另有楔形细胞（3）及未分化细胞等类型。固有层由成纤维细胞（4）、胶原（5）和毛细血管等组成。

HPM: Figure 18-2b shows the mucosal columnar epithelium of the fallopian tube consisting of two cell types. The ciliated cells (1) with apical cilia that beat toward the uterus. The fewer secretory cells (2) are non-ciliated. There are also other cell types, such as wedge cells (3), undifferentiated cells. The lamina propria consists of fibroblast cells (4), collagens (5), and capillaries.

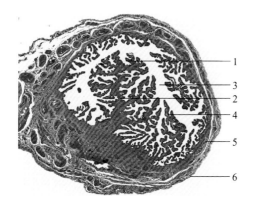

图 18-2a 输卵管（20×）

Fig. 18-2a Fallopian tube (20×)

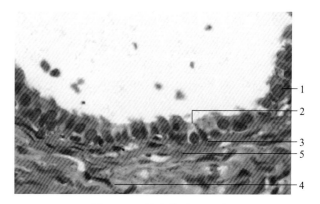

图 18-2b 输卵管（400×）

Fig. 18-2b Fallopian tube (400×)

❸ 切片 3：子宫

材料与方法：人的子宫，HE 染色。

低倍镜观察：图 18-3a 显示子宫壁由子宫内膜（1）、肌层（2）和外膜组成。子宫内膜由表面的单层柱状上皮（3）和固有层组成。固有层内含有腺体（4）、基质以及螺旋动脉等结构。肌层由三层分界不明显的平滑肌组成。子宫外膜在子宫底部与体部为浆膜，其余部位为纤维膜。

3. Section 3: Uterus

Materials and methods: Uterus of human, paraffin embedding, HE staining.

LPM: Figure 18-3a shows the uterus, which consists of the endometrium (1), myometrium (2), and perimetrium. The endometrium consists of simple columnar epithelium (3) and the lamina propria, which consists of glands (4), stoma and spiral arterials. The myometrium consists of three indistinct layers of smooth muscle. The perimetrium of uterus is serosa membrane at the bottom and body of the uterus, but is fibrous membrane at the rest part.

高倍镜观察：图 18-3b 显示子宫内膜固有层基质（1）内可见基质细胞，子宫腺体（2）的腺上皮由单层腺上皮细胞组成。增殖期腺体较少，短而直；间质疏松。间质内可见较多螺旋小动脉（3）。

HPM: Figure 18-3b shows lamina propria (1), in which stromal cells can be seen. The glandular epithelium of uterus glands (2) consists of simple layer glandular epithelial cells. The glands in proliferative phase are fewer, short and straight. The mesenchyma is loose, with numerous spiral arterials (3).

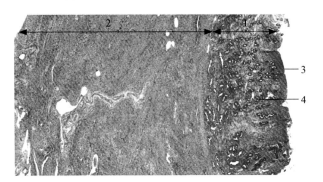 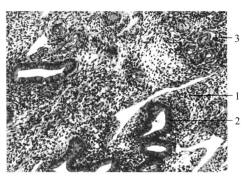

图 18-3a　子宫（20×）

Fig. 18-3a　Uterus (20×)

图 18-3b　子宫内膜增殖期（200×）

Fig. 18-3b　Uterus endometrium on proliferative phase (200×)

④ 切片 4：子宫内膜分泌期

材料与方法：人子宫内膜，HE 染色。

低倍镜观察：图 18-4 显示分泌期子宫内膜，此时子宫内膜厚度增加，子宫腺体（1）增长、弯曲，腺腔扩大，腺腔内可见分泌物。间质水肿，螺旋小动脉（2）增多。

4. Section 4: Secretory uterus endometrium

Materials and methods: uterus of human, paraffin embedding, HE staining.

LPM: Figure 18-4 shows the uterus endometrium in secretary phase, which is characterized by thickened endometrium, lengthened and curved endometrial glands (1), enlarged endometrial lumen with secretion products. In addition, interstitial edema and increased spiral arterials (2) can be observed.

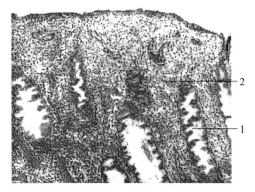

图 18-4　子宫内膜分泌期（100×）

Fig. 18-4　Uterus endometrium in secretory phase (100×)

⑤ 切片 5：子宫颈

材料与方法：人子宫颈，HE 染色。

低倍镜观察：图 18-5a 显示子宫颈黏膜上皮分成两种类型：宫颈管黏膜（1）（宫颈内、外口之间）表面的单层柱状上皮，宫颈外口（2）到阴道穹隆（3）之间的复层鳞状上皮（4）。宫颈上皮在固有层下陷成腺样隐窝，称为子宫颈腺（5）。两种类型的上皮交接处（6）是宫颈癌好发部位。肌层（7）大致为内环外纵的平滑肌不规则排列所成。

5. Section 5: Cervix

Materials and Methods: Cervix of human, paraffin embedding, HE staining.

LPM: Figure 18-5a shows the cervical mucosa which consists of two types of cervical mucosal epithelium, the single layer of columnar epithelium on the surface of the cervical duct mucosa (1)

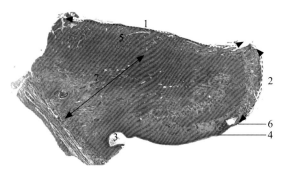

图 18-5a　子宫颈（40×）（图片由山东数字人提供）
Fig. 18-5a　Cervix (40×) (This figure is provided by Shandong Digihuman Technology Co., Inc)

(between the inside and outside of the cervix), and the stratified squamous epithelium (4) between the outer cervix (2) and the vaginal fornix (3). The glands in the lamina propria is called cervical gland (5). The epithelial junction (6) between two types of cells is the most common site for cervical cancer. The muscular layer (7) roughly consists of inner circular and outer longitudinal smooth muscles in irregular arrangement.

高倍镜观察：图 18-5b 显示子宫颈复层鳞状上皮（1）与单层柱状上皮（2）的移行部位（3）（注：本图移行部位可见部分柱状上皮鳞状化生现象），（4）为宫颈腺。图 18-5c 显示子宫颈单层高柱状上皮细胞（1）。

HPM: Figure 18-5b shows the transitional site (3) between the cervical stratified squamous epithelium (1) and the single columnar epithelium (2). (Note: The squamous metaplasia of partial columnar epithelium is seen at the transitional site.) The cervical gland shows as (4). Figure 18-5c shows the cervical single layer tall columnar epithelial cells (1).

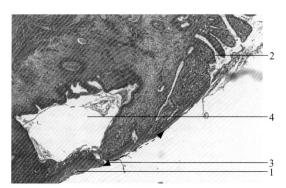

图 18-5b　子宫颈上皮移行（100×）
Fig. 18-5b　Transformation zone of cervical epithelium (100×)

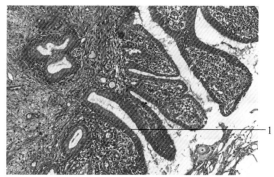

图 18-5c　子宫颈柱状上皮（200×）
Fig. 18-5c　Cervical columnar epithelium (200×)

❻ 切片 6：乳腺（静止期）

材料与方法：人乳腺，HE 染色。

低倍镜观察：图 18-6a 显示乳腺的大部分区域为结缔组织（1），可见较多的胶原纤维，也可见血管和脂肪组织（2）等。乳腺小叶（3）很分散，由腺泡、导管和结缔组织组成。导管（4）包括小叶内导管、小叶间导管和总导管。

6. Section 6: Mammary gland (stationary phase)

Materials and methods: Mammary gland of human, paraffin embedding, HE staining.

LPM: Figure 18-6a shows that the majority part of mammary gland is connective tissue (1), in which collagens, blood vessels and adipose tissue (2) etc. can be observed. The scattered mammary lobules (3) consist of acini, ducts and connective tissues. The ducts (4) include intralobular ducts, interlobular ducts and lactiferous ducts.

高倍镜观察：图 18-6b 显示乳腺腺泡上皮（1）为单层立方或柱状，在上皮细胞和基膜（2）间有肌上皮细胞（3）。腺泡有腔（4）或无腔。毛细血管（5），成纤维细胞（6）以及胶原束（7）可见。

HPM: Figure 18-6b shows the epithelium (1) of mammary glands consisting of simple cuboidal or columnar epithelial cells. The myoepithelial cells (3) exist between glandular epithelium and basement membrane (2). The acini are shown with or without lumen (4). Capillaries (5), fibroblasts (6), and collagen bundles (7) can be seen.

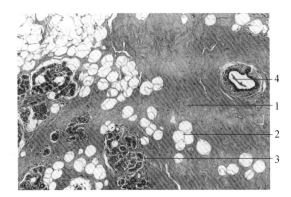

图 18-6a 乳腺静止期（100×）

Fig. 18-6a Resting mammary gland (100×)

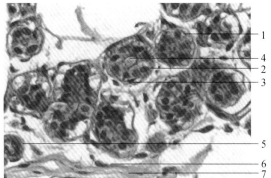

图 18-6b 乳腺静止期（400×）

Fig. 18-6b Resting mammary gland (400×)

❼ 切片 7：乳腺（分泌期）

材料与方法：人乳腺，HE 染色。

低倍镜观察：图 18-7a 显示分泌期的乳腺。小导管（1）和腺泡（2），迅速增生增大，结缔组织和脂肪组织相应减少。腔内含有乳汁分泌物（3）。

7. Section 7: Mammary gland (secretory phase)

Materials and methods: Mammary gland of human, paraffin embedding, HE staining.

LPM: Figure 18-7a shows the secretory mammary gland. The small ducts (1) and acini (2) proliferate and enlarge rapidly. Connective tissue and adipose tissue decrease. The glandular lumens contain milk secretion (3).

高倍镜观察：图 18-7b 显示乳腺的腺泡上皮（1）呈单层柱状或立方上皮，腺泡腔增大，腔内充满乳汁（2），染成红色的部分为乳汁中的蛋白成分，空泡是乳汁中的脂滴溶解而成。

HPM: Figure 18-7b shows the acinar epithelium (1) composed of simple columnar or cuboidal cells. The acinar lumens enlarge and contain milk (2) . The red-stained part is protein component of milk, and the vesicular part is dissolved lipid droplet.

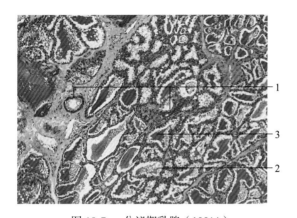

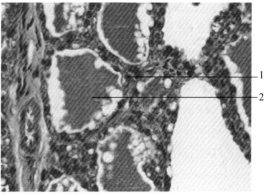

图 18-7a　分泌期乳腺（100×）

Fig. 18-7a　Secretory mammary gland（100×）

图 18-7b　分泌期乳腺（400×）

Fig. 18-7b　Secretory mammary gland（400×）

【示教切片】
【Teaching Sections】

⑧ 切片 8：妊娠黄体

材料与方法：人的卵巢，HE 染色。

低倍镜观察：图 18-8a 显示妊娠黄体（1）体积很大，外被结缔组织被膜，与周围组织分界清楚。妊娠期间的卵泡（2）多处于闭锁状态。

8. Section 8: Corpora luteum of pregnancy

Materials and methods: the ovary of human, paraffin embedding, HE staining.

LPM: Figure 18-8a shows a corpus luteum (1) of pregnancy. It is large, covered by connective tissue capsule, separated clearly from the surrounding tissue. During pregnancy, the follicles (2) are mostly atretic follicles.

高倍镜观察：图 18-8b 显示妊娠黄体内，颗粒黄体细胞（1）体积大，多边形，核圆形，核仁清楚，胞质色浅。膜黄体细胞（2）体积较小，形态不规则，着色较深，位于靠近结缔

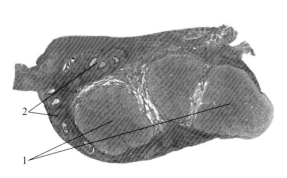

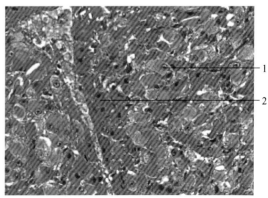

图 18-8a　妊娠黄体（50×）

Fig. 18-8a　Corpus luteum of pregnancy（50×）

图 18-8b　妊娠黄体（400×）

Fig. 18-8b　Corpus luteum of pregnancy（400×）

组织隔的部位。

HPM: Figure 18-8b shows a corpus luteum of pregnancy. The granulosa lutein cells (1) are larger, polygonal. They have spherical nuclei, distinct nucleoli, and pale staining cytoplasm. The theca lutein cells (2) are smaller, irregular shape, with deeper staining cytoplasm, and are located close to the connective tissue septa.

【作业】

绘图描述成熟卵泡的组织结构。

【Assignment】

Please draw the histological structure of mature follicle.

【思考题】

1. 描述卵巢各阶段卵泡的生长、发育及成熟的结构特点。
2. 试述黄体的形成、形态结构及功能。

【Questions】

1. Please describe the morphological features of the ovarian follicles on the growth, development and mature stages.

2. Please describe the formation, structure and function of corpora luteum.

【临床与科研联系英文阅读材料】
【English Reading Material for Correlations with Clinic and Scientific Research】

Nearly 90% of ovarian malignancies are epithelial ovarian carcinomas arising from the ovarian surface (germinal) epithelium. Ovarian cancer is one of the most common gynecologic cancers and the fifth most frequent cause of death in women. The risk of ovarian cancer increases with age, and occurs mostly in postmenopausal women. About 10% of ovarian cancers are familial, three distinct hereditary patterns having been identified. In most families affected by the breast and ovarian cancer syndrome, a genetic linkage on the BRCA1 locus of chromosome 17q21 has been found. Ovarian cancer usually spreads by local shedding into the peritoneal cavity followed by implantation in the peritoneal surface.

（王大亮）

第 19 章 眼 和 耳

Chapter 19 Eye and Ear

【实习内容】Contents of Observation

切片 Sections

1. 眼球	1. Eyeball
2. 内耳	2. Inner ear

【目的要求】

1. 掌握眼球壁的组织结构（重点为角膜、虹膜、睫状体及视网膜）。
2. 了解螺旋器的组织结构。

【Objective】

1. To master the structural characteristics of the wall of eyeball, especially cornea, iris, ciliary body and retina.

2. To understand morphological features of the organ of Corti.

【观察切片】
【Observation Sections】

1 切片 1：眼球

材料与方法：人眼球，HE 染色。

低倍镜观察：

（1）眼球壁

图 19-1a 眼球壁由外层的纤维膜、中间的血管膜和内层的视网膜构成。纤维膜由前部的

角膜（1）和后部的巩膜（2）构成，两者移行处称角膜缘（3）；血管膜分为三部分：虹膜（4）、脉络膜（5）、睫状体（6）；视网膜由视网膜视部和视网膜盲部构成。

1. Section 1: Eyeball

Materials and methods: Human eyeball, HE staining.

LPM：

(1) Wall of eyeball

Figure 19-1a shows that the wall of eyebau has three tissue layers, the outer fibrous tunica,

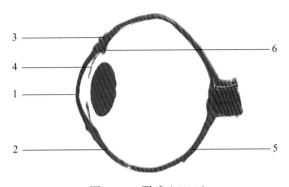

图 19-1a　眼球（40×）
Fig. 19-1a　Eyeball（40×）

the middle vascular tunica and the inner retina. Fibrous tunica consists of anterior cornea (1) and posterior sclera (2), and the transitional area called corneoscleral limbus (3). Vascular tunica consists of iris (4), choroid (5) and ciliary body (6). Retina consists of nonneural region and neural retina.

高倍镜观察：

（2）眼球前部

1）角膜：由前向后分为5层：角膜上皮层（1）、前界层（2）、角膜基质（3）、后界层（4）以及角膜内皮（5）（图 19-1b）。

HPM：

(2) Anterior part of eyeball

1) Cornea consists of corneal epithelium (1), anterior limiting lamina (2), corneal stroma (3), posterior limiting lamina (4) and corneal endothelium (5) (Figure 19-1b).

2）前房角：为角膜与虹膜的夹角（图 19-1c）。

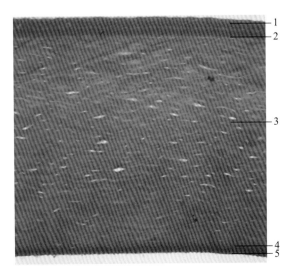

图 19-1b　角膜（200×）
Fig. 19-1b　Cornea（200×）

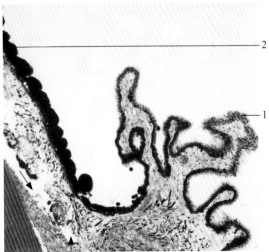

图 19-1c　前房角与睫状体（400×）
Fig. 19-1c　Angle of anterior chamber and Ciliary body（400×）

2) Angle of the anterior chamber is at the junction of the cornea and base of iris (Figure 19-1c).

3）睫状体：睫状体内侧有睫状突（1），睫状突上皮由两层细胞构成，外层的非色素上皮细胞和内层的色素细胞。同时可以观察到虹膜（2）（图 19-1c）。

3) Ciliary body: The inner surface of Ciliary body has ciliary processes (1), which consists of double-layered epithelium, the outer nonpigmented epithelial layer and the inner pigmented epithelial layer. The iris also can be seen (2) (Figure 19-1c).

4）虹膜：位于角膜和晶状体之间，根部与睫状体相连，中央为瞳孔。由前缘层（1）（不连续成纤维细胞和色素细胞）、虹膜基质（2）以及虹膜上皮层（3）（表层立方形色素上皮和深层肌上皮细胞特化为瞳孔括约肌和瞳孔开大肌）构成（图 19-1d）。

4) Iris is between the cornea and lens. Its root is in continuity with the ciliary body. Its central adjustable aperture is the pupil. Iris consists of anterior surface (1) (discontinuous layer of fibroblasts and pigmented melanocytes); Iris stroma (2), and Iris epithelium (3) (superficial layer of pigmented cuboidal epithelium and inner layer of myoepithelial cells that forms the dilator pupillae muscle and constrictor pupillae muscle) (Figure 19-1d).

（3）眼球后部

包括致密结缔组织组成的巩膜，富有大量色素细胞及血管的脉络膜以及视网膜（由外向内观察）。

(3) Posterior part of eye

Posterior part of the eye includes sclera that consists of dense connective tissue; choroid that is rich in pigment cells and blood vessels and retina.

1）视网膜视部：通常所指的视网膜，可辨认 10 层结构（图 19-1e）：色素上皮层（1）、视杆视锥层（2）、外界膜（3）、外胞核层（4）、外网织层（5）、内胞核层（6）、内网织层

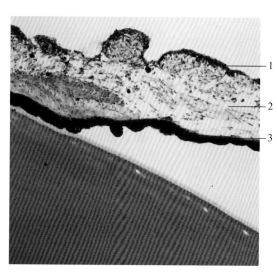

图 19-1d　虹膜（400×）
Fig. 19-1d　Iris (400×)

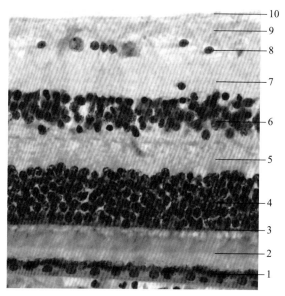

图 19-1e　视网膜视部 10 层结构模式图（400×）
Fig. 19-1e　Ten layers of retina (400×)

（7）、节细胞层（8）、视神经纤维层（9）、和内界膜（10）。

1) Visual part of the retina, commonly referred to as the retina. Ten layers of retina can be distinguished (Figure 19-1e): the pigment epithelium (1), rods and cones (2), external limiting membrane (3), outer nuclear layer (4), outer plexiform layer (5), inner nuclear layer (6), inner plexiform layer (7), ganglion cell layer (8), nerve fiber layer (9), and the internal limiting membrane (10).

2）锯齿缘（图 19-1f）：视网膜视部，即神经部（1），向前与视网膜盲部，即非神经部（2），相连，两者交界处参差不齐，称锯齿缘（3）。此处视网膜常因制作标本时有剥脱而呈隆起状，此处也是临床上视网膜剥脱处。

2) Ora serrata (Figure 19-1f) (3) is a ragged margin between neural (1) and non-neural parts (2) of the retina. Separation at this site is a common artifact of preparation; however, clinically this is also a common site of retinal detachment.

3）视神经乳头（视盘）（箭头）：为视神经纤维集中走出巩膜处（图 19-1g）。

3) Papilla of optic nerve (optic disc) (arrow) : is the exit site of the optic nerve that penetrates the sclera (Figure 19-1g).

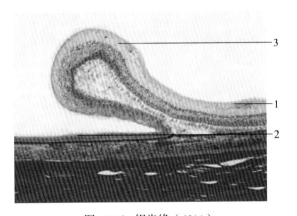

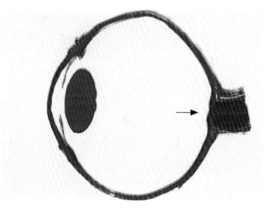

图 19-1f 锯齿缘（40×）
Fig. 19-1f Ora serrate (40×)

图 19-1g 神经乳头（视盘）（40×）
Fig. 19-1g Papilla of optic nerve (optic disc) (40×)

4）黄斑：位于眼球的后极，其中央有一凹陷称中央凹（箭头），主要含有色素上皮和视锥细胞。此处无血管（图 19-1h）。

4) Macula lutea: lies at the posterior pole of the eye. In the center of the macula lutea is fovea

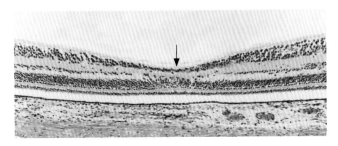

图 19-1h 黄斑的中央凹（100×）
Fig. 19-1h Central fovea of the macula lutea (100×)

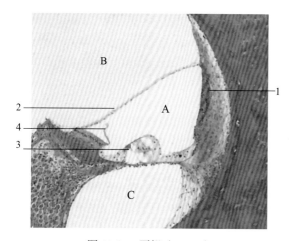

图 19-2a　耳蜗（100×）

Fig. 19-2a　Cochlea (100×)

centralis (arrow). Fovea centralis shows markedly attenuated retinal layer, with no blood vessels and almost all photoreceptors are tightly packed cones (Figure 19-1h).

② 切片2：内耳

材料与方法：豚鼠内耳，HE 染色。

高倍镜观察：

耳蜗：耳蜗被分成三部分（图 19-2a）：膜蜗管（A），螺旋板上外侧的三角形腔；前庭阶（B），位于膜蜗管上面；鼓室阶（C），位于膜蜗管下面。膜蜗管外侧为血管纹（1），富含血管的假复层上皮，分泌内淋巴。前庭膜（2），位于膜蜗管的顶端，由两层单层扁平上皮细胞构成，与前庭阶相隔。基膜，位于膜蜗管的底端，较厚，与鼓室阶相隔。基膜上是高度特异的上皮，Corti 器（即螺旋器）（3）：由毛细胞和支持细胞构成。毛细胞是特异的听觉感受细胞，游离面有静纤毛，静纤毛顶端嵌入凝胶状的盖膜（4）上。Corti 器底端与传入神经纤维末梢形成突触。

2. Section 2: Inner ear

Materials and methods: Inner ear of guinea pig, HE staining.

HPM:

Cochlea: has a lumen with three compartments (Figure 19-2a): cochlear duct (A), a triangle space in transverse section, scala vestibuli (B) above the cochlear duct, and scala tympani (C) under the cochlear duct. Lateral border of cochlear duct makes up the stria vascularis (1) a richly vascularized pseudostratified epithelium, that secretes endolymph. Vestibular membrane (2), which marks the roof of the cochlear duct, consists of two layers of simple squamous epithelium and delineates cochlear duct from scala vestibuli. A thicker basilar membrane forms the floor of the cochlear duct and separates it from scala tympani. Superimposed on the basilar membrane is highly specialized epithelium, the organ of Corti (spiral organ) (3), which consists of hair cells and supporting cells. Cochlear hair cells are specialized auditory receptor cells. They have apical stereocilia, whose tips are embedded in the gelatinous tectorial membrane (4). Arising from the base of the organ of Corti are afferent nerve fibers that synapse with the base of hair cells.

科尔蒂器（图 19-2b）基膜（1）上有三排外毛细胞（2）和一排内毛细胞（3）。外毛细胞顶端静纤毛顶端嵌入盖膜（4）。薄而倾斜的前庭膜将前庭阶内的外淋巴与膜蜗管内的内淋巴分隔。

Organ of Corti (Figure 19-2b): On the basilar membrane (1), there are three rows of outer hair cells (2) and a row of inner hair cells (3). Apical stereocilia of outer hair cells protrude into the tectorial membrane (4). A thin, slanting vestibular membrane separates perilymph in the scala vestibule from endolymph in the cochlear duct.

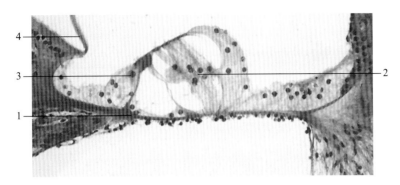

图 19-2b　科尔蒂器（400×）

Fig. 19-2b　Organ of Corti (400×)

【思考题】

简述角膜的组织结构及其透明的主要因素。

【Questions】

Describe the structural features and the main factors for the transparency of the cornea.

【临床与科研联系英文阅读材料】
【English Reading Material for Correlations with Clinic and Scientific Research】

Meniere's disease is a disorder of the inner ear. It can cause severe dizziness, a roaring sound in your ears called tinnitus, hearing loss that comes and goes and the feeling of ear pressure or pain. It usually affects just one ear. It is a common cause of hearing loss.

Attacks of dizziness may come suddenly or after a short period of tinnitus or muffled hearing. Some people have single attacks of dizziness occasionally. Others may have many attacks closing together over several days. Some people with Meniere's disease have "drop attacks" during which the dizziness is so bad that they lose their balance and fall.

Scientists do not yet know the cause. They think that it has to do with the fluid levels or the mixing of fluids in the canals of your inner ear. Diagnosis of this disease is based on physical exam and your symptoms. A hearing test can be done to check how it has affected your hearing.

There is no cure. Treatments include medications to control dizziness, limiting salt in your diet, and taking water pills. A device that fits into the outer ear and delivers air pulses to the middle ear can be helpful. Severe cases may require surgery.

（任彩霞）

思考题答案要点

Key Points of Questions

第1章 细　　胞

答题要点：

1. 主要细胞器以及其主要功能：

1）线粒体：由两层膜包被的细胞器，主要功能是真核生物进行氧化磷酸化合成 ATP，为细胞直接提供能量。

2）核糖体：在细胞中负责由 RNA 到蛋白质这一过程，是细胞内合成蛋白质的场所。

3）内质网：

a. 粗面内质网：主要功能是合成分泌蛋白质、溶酶体蛋白和部分膜蛋白等。

b. 滑面内质网：滑面内质网的功能多种多样，主要参与合成类固醇激素、解毒功能以及离子的储存和释放等。

4）高尔基体：将内质网合成的蛋白质进行加工、修饰、浓缩和糖基化，最终形成分泌颗粒并排到细胞外。

5）溶酶体：是细胞内消化作用的主要场所。

2. 细胞骨架：指真核细胞中的蛋白纤维网络结构。主要包括微管、微丝及中间纤维。

1）微管：在细胞形态的形成和维持中起重要作用，并参与细胞的运动以及细胞内细胞器小泡的运输。

2）微丝：与微管和中间纤维共同组成细胞骨架并参与细胞运动。

3）中间纤维：是最稳定的细胞骨架成分，它主要起支撑作用。

3. 常染色质：呈松散状，染色较浅而均匀，含有单一或重复序列的 DNA，具有转录活性；异染色质：呈凝集状态，螺旋化程度较高，而且染色较深，含有重复 DNA 序列，很少进行转录或无转录活性。

4. 细胞周期包括：分为间期与分裂期两个阶段。间期又分为三期，即 G_1（DNA 合成前期）、S 期（DNA 合成期）与 G_2 期（DNA 合成后期）；M 期：细胞分裂期。

Chapter 1　Cell

Answer points:

1. The basal cytoplasmic organelles and their functions:

1) Mitochondria: Mitochondria are organelles coated by two layers of membrane, the main function of which is the oxidative phosphorylation in eukaryotes to generate ATP to provide direct energy for the eukaryotic cell.

2) Ribosome: The ribosome is responsible for the process from RNA to protein in eukaryotic cells. It is the site for protein synthesis in cells.

3) Endoplasmic reticulum:

a. Rough endoplasmic reticulum (RER): Its main function is to synthesize and secrete proteins, lysosomal proteins, and some membrane proteins etc.

b. Smooth endoplasmic reticulum (SER): SER has various functions. SER is involved in the synthesis of steroid hormones, detoxification functions, and storage and release of ions etc.

4) Golgi apparatus: The proteins synthesized by the endoplasmic reticulum are processed, modified, concentrated and glycosylated in Golgi apparatus for secretion.

5) Lysosomes: Lysosomes are sites of intracellular digestion.

2. Cytoskeleton: It is a complex network, consisting of protein microtubules (MT), microfilaments (MF) and intermediate filaments (IF).

1) MT: The cytoplasmic microtubules play a significant role in the formation and maintenance of cell shape, and participate in the movement of cells and the transport of cell organelle vesicles within cells.

2) MF: Microfilaments together with microtubules and intermediate fibers form the cytoskeleton and are involved in the cell movement.

3) IF: The most stable cytoskeleton component, which plays a major role in supporting.

3. Euchromatin is the less coiled portion of chromosomes, visible as lightly and uniformly stained areas, and contains both non-repeated and repeated sequence of DNA, which has transcriptional activity.

Heterochromatin is tightly packaged, with a high degree of helix and deep staining. Heterochromatin contains repeated DNA sequences and is transcriptional inactive.

4. The Cell cycle includes interphase and mitosis. The interphase has three distinct periods termed G_1 (the gap between mitosis and DNA replication), S (the period of DNA synthesis), and G_2 (the gap between DNA replication and the next mitosis). M phase is the mitotic period.

第 2 章　上 皮 组 织

答题要点：

1. 游离面和基底面。游离面：细胞衣、微绒毛和纤毛；基底面：基膜、质膜内褶和半桥粒。

2. 由柱状细胞、梭形细胞、锥体细胞和杯状细胞组成，柱状细胞游离面有纤毛。细胞高矮不等，细胞核的位置也不在同一水平，但所有细胞的基底部均附着于基膜上。主要分布在呼吸道表面。

3. 分布部位不同。复层扁平上皮表面有数层扁平状细胞，核小染色深；中层为多边形或梭形细胞；上皮与深层结缔组织的连接面呈凹凸不平波浪状。皮肤表皮的复层扁平上皮浅层可见角质层。变移上皮细胞形状和层数随所在器官的功能状况改变而变化，表层细胞较大，一个细胞常覆盖其深面几个细胞，核染色较浅，可见核仁。

Chapter 2   Epithelial Tissue

Answer points:

1. The epithelial cell has apical surface and basal surface.

On apical surface: cell coat, microvillus, and cilium.

On basal surface: basement membrane, plasma membrane infolding, and hemidesmosome.

2. Pseudostratified ciliated columnar epithelium is composed of columnar cells, goblet cells, fusiform cells and cone cells. Cilia can be found on the apical surface of columnar cells. The epithelial cells are different in height, thus the nuclei of cells are disposed at different levels. But all the cells rest on the basement membrane. Pseudostratified ciliated columnar epithelium is found in the lining of respiratory tract.

3. The distributions of stratified squamous epithelium and transitional epithelium are different. The surface layer of stratified squamous epithelium has several layers of flatten cells, with small and dark-staining nuclei. The intermediate layer contains polygonal or fusiform cells. The basal surface of the epithelium is irregular and wavy. In epidermis, the superficial portion of stratified squamous epithelium is keratinized. In transitional epithelium, the layer and shape of epithelial cells can change according to the organ function. The superficial cells are large, with light-staining nucleus and prominent nucleolus.

第 3 章　结　缔　组　织

答题要点：

1. 光镜下细胞呈圆形或卵圆形，大小不等，细胞质强嗜碱性，近核周有浅染区域即核周晕。细胞核圆形，常偏位，染色质致密，呈辐射状排列。电镜下可见大量平行排列的粗面内质网，核周晕区有发达的高尔基复合体和中心体。

2. 光镜下成纤维细胞呈扁平星状，多突起；细胞质丰富，弱嗜碱性；细胞核椭圆形，染色浅，核仁明显。电镜下可见丰富的粗面内质网，游离核糖体和发达的高尔基复合体。纤维细胞是功能不活跃状态的成纤维细胞，体积小，细胞扁平或梭形，细胞核小，染色深，细胞质少，弱嗜酸性。电镜下粗面内质网少，高尔基复合体不发达。

Chapter 3   Connective Tissue

Answer points:

1. The typically mature plasma cells are oval; their cytoplasm is deeply basophilic; a clear area near the eccentric, round nucleus is a juxtanuclear halo (negative Golgi image), which corresponds to the Golgi complex; The nuclear chromatin is mostly condensed and heterochromatic, alternating with light areas, to give a spoke-wheel or clock-face appearance.

2. Fibroblasts are ovoid or stellate cells with long, tapering processes that branch. They have one

elliptical nucleus, usually euchromatic, with one or more distinct nucleoli. Light microscopy shows that staining attributes of their cytoplasm differ according to their functional state. Active or immature cells have weakly basophilic, relatively conspicuous cytoplasm. Mature or inactive cells (fibrocytes) have weakly acidophilic, barely visible cytoplasm with a relatively homogeneous appearance. Electron microscopic features of fibroblasts are typical of most protein-synthesizing cells.

第 4 章　软　骨　与　骨

答题要点:

1. 间骨板形成: 是原有的环骨板和骨单位因骨组织增长或改建被破坏吸收而残留的部分。

2. 软骨囊与软骨陷窝: 两者不是同一结构。软骨囊是紧靠软骨细胞周围的软骨间质。HE 染色时, 因为其内含较多的硫酸软骨素而嗜碱性强, 呈蓝色。软骨陷窝不是软骨基质, 而是其内容纳软骨细胞的空间。

Chapter 4　Cartilage and Bone

Answer points:

1. The formation of interstitial lamella: During the bone growth or rebuilding, the osteon is broken. After absorption of some osseous tissue, the residual fraction becomes interstitial lamella.

2. Cartilage capsule and cartilage lacuna: They are not the same structure. Cartilage capsule is the cartilage matrix just around the chondrocyte. Because of lots of chondroitin sulfate, it is strong basophilic and dark blue after H.E. staining. Cartilage lacuna is not a part of the cartilage matrix, but just a space in it holding the chondrocyte.

第 5 章　血液和血细胞的发生

答题要点:

中性粒细胞, 形态不规则, 外周常有突起, 胞质淡红色。细胞内含许多弥散分布的细小的浅红或浅紫色的特有颗粒。这些颗粒多是溶酶体, 颗粒中含有过氧化物酶、酸性磷酸酶、吞噬素、溶菌酶等, 与细胞的吞噬和消化功能有关。细胞核呈杆状或 2～5 分叶状, 叶与叶间有细丝相连。主要功能:

1)趋化作用: 中性粒细胞在化学趋向因子的作用下, 可向目的物移行。炎症时, 在化学趋向因子的作用下, 粒细胞先吸附于血管壁, 然后向血管外移行至组织。

2)调理素作用: 血清调理素在免疫球蛋白和补体参与下, 可使微生物吸附于粒细胞膜上, 进而发挥吞噬作用。

3)吞噬作用: 经调理素作用后, 吸附于粒细胞膜上的微生物被粒细胞伸出的伪足包围, 胞膜凹陷形成空泡, 称为吞噬体。

4)脱粒作用: 粒细胞细胞质内含有嗜天青颗粒和特异性颗粒, 嗜天青颗粒内含过氧化物酶、中性酸性水解酶和溶菌酶等, 特异性颗粒除含有溶菌酶外, 还含有胶原酶、溶酶体和碱性磷酸酶。细胞质颗粒可进入吞噬体内, 释放出各种酶类以杀灭细菌。

5)杀菌作用: 粒细胞经吞噬作用后发生代谢变化, 耗氧增加, 过氧化氢产生增多, 磷酸戊糖旁路代谢增强，部分过氧化氢进入吞噬空泡，与过氧化物酶作用后起杀菌作用。

Chapter 5　Blood and Hematopoiesis

Answer points:

Neutrophils are irregular in shape, often protruding at the periphery and have pale red cytoplasm. The cells contain many scattered small red or light purple special granules. Most of these granules are lysosomes, which contain peroxidase, acid phosphatase, phagocytin, and lysozyme and so on. They are important in phagocytosis and digestion of cells. The nucleus is rod-shaped or divided into 2-5 lobes, which are connected by thin strings in between. Main functions:

1) Chemotaxis: neutrophils can migrate to the target under the action of chemotactic factors. In inflammation, under the action of chemotactic factors, granulocytes first adhere to the vessel wall, and then migrate to the tissue outside the blood vessels.

2) Opsonization: serum immunoglobulin and complements participate in the adsorption of microbes to the granulocyte membrane to be ingested by the granulocytes. .

3) Phagocytosis: after the action of opsonization, the microorganism adsorbed on the membrane of the granulocyte is surrounded by the protruding periphery part of the granulocyte, and the vacuoles are formed by the cell membrane, forming phagocytic vacuoles called phagosomes .

4) Fusion of phagosome with lysosome: the cytoplasm of granulocyte contains eosinophilic granules and specific particles. The eosinophilic granules contain peroxidase, neutral acid hydrolase and lysozyme. The specific particles contain collagenase, lysosome and alkaline phosphatase in addition to lysozyme. Those cytoplasm particles can fuse with the phagosomes to become phagolysosomes and release various enzymes to kill the engulfed microorganisms. Since all these killing mechanisms are normally sequestered in phagolysosomes, to which phagocytosed materials are brought, the potentially harmful substances are therefore segregated from the cell's cytoplasm and nucleus to avoid damage to the phagocyte while it is performing its normal function.

5) Bactericidal effect: after the granulocyte phagocytosis, a series of metabolic changes happen, including oxygen consumption increased, hydrogen peroxide production increased, pentose phosphate bypass increased, some hydrogen peroxide into the phagolysosomes to kill or degrade the ingested material under the action of peroxidase.

第 6 章　肌　组　织

答题要点：

1. 肌组织几乎都是由肌细胞或者肌纤维组成。可分为三种：

1）平滑肌：纤维呈长梭形，无横纹，每个细胞一个核。

2）骨骼肌：呈纤维状，有明显横纹，核多且都位于细胞膜下方。

3）心肌：有横纹，为短柱状，一般只有一个细胞核。心肌细胞之间有闰盘结构。

2. 骨骼肌的横纹是由明带和暗带组成；心肌纤维的横纹除了明带和暗带，还有闰盘结构。

3. 骨骼肌由肌纤维组成，每条肌纤维由粗肌丝与细肌丝相对滑动而使肌肉收缩，产生运动。骨骼肌收缩的机制是肌丝滑动原理。其过程大致如下：

1）运动神经末梢将神经冲动传递给肌膜；

2）肌膜的兴奋经横小管迅速传向终池；

3）肌浆网膜上的钙泵活动，将大量 Ca^{2+} 转运到肌浆内；

4）肌原蛋白 TnC 与 Ca^{2+} 结合后，发生构型改变，进而使原肌球蛋白位置也随之变化，原来被掩盖的肌动蛋白位点暴露，迅即与肌球蛋白头接触；

5）肌球蛋白头 ATP 酶被激活，分解了 ATP 并释放能量；

6）肌球蛋白的头及杆发生屈曲转动，将肌动蛋白拉向 M 线；

7）细肌丝向 A 带内滑入，I 带变窄，A 带长度不变，但 H 带因细肌丝的插入可消失，由于细肌丝在粗肌丝之间向 M 线滑动，肌节缩短，肌纤维收缩；

8）收缩完毕，肌浆内 Ca^{2+} 被泵入肌浆网内，肌浆内 Ca^{2+} 浓度降低，肌原蛋白恢复原来构型，原肌球蛋白恢复原位又掩盖肌动蛋白位点，肌球蛋白头与肌动蛋白脱离接触，肌则处于松弛状态。

4．心肌纤维之间通过闰盘连接，主要是传导兴奋的作用。

Chapter 6　　Muscle Tissue

Answer points:

1. Muscle tissue are composed of muscle cells or muscle fibers, muscle tissue can be divided into three types.

1) Smooth muscle: Smooth muscle consists of collections of fusiform cells that do not show striations, and each cell has a single nucleus.

2) Skeletal muscle: Skeletal muscle is composed of bundles of very long, cylindrical, multinucleated cells that show cross striations. The long oval nuclei are usually found at the periphery of the cell under cell membrane.

3) Cardiac muscle: Cardiac muscle has cross striations and is composed of elongated, branched individual cells that lie parallel to each other. The intercalated disk structures are found only in cardiac muscle.

2. The cross striations of skeletal muscle are composed of alternating light and dark bands.

3. The mechanism of skeletal muscle contraction is filament sliding. The process is as follows:

1) The endings of the motor nerve transfer the impulses to the myolemma;

2) The impulse of the myolemma quickly passes through T tubule to the terminal pool;

3) The calcium pump is activated by the dissemination of the impulses to release a large number of Ca^{2+} concentrated within the lumen of the sarcoplasmic reticulum into the sarcoplasm surrounding the myofilaments;

4) Combining with Ca^{2+}, results in the configuration change of Troponin TnC, and the change of position of tropomyosin actin: the original concealed site is exposed and is in immediate contact with the myosin head;

5) ATP enzyme of myosin head is activated. ATP is used to release energy;

6) The head and rod of myosin is flexed, and actin is pulled to the M line;

7) Thin filaments slide to A band, I band becomes narrower, while A band length unchanged. Due to the insertion of thin filaments, H band can disappear. Because the thin filaments slide to the M line between the thick filaments, sarcomere shortens and muscle fiber contracts.

8) After contracting, calcium in the sarcoplasm are pumped into the sarcoplasmic reticulum, the Ca^{2+} concentration in the sarcoplasm decreases, the myofibril returns to its original configuration, and the tropomyosin resumes its original position to cover the actin site. The myosin head is isolated from the actin, and the muscle is in a relaxed state.

4. The intercalated disc connection among the cardiac muscle fibers is mainly to conduct excitation.

第 7 章　神 经 组 织

答题要点：

1. 多极神经元有一个轴突和两个或者多个树突。如脊髓前角运动神经元，胞体大，有一个轴突和多个树突，胞体内有尼氏体。

2. 神经胶质细胞：星形胶质细胞、少突胶质细胞、小胶质细胞、室管膜细胞；周围神经系统胶质细胞：施万细胞、卫星细胞。

3. 神经末梢：根据功能不同分为感觉神经末梢和运动神经末梢。感觉神经末梢又分为游离神经末梢、有被囊神经末梢。有被囊神经末梢有触觉小体、环层小体以及肌梭。运动神经末梢又分为躯体及内脏运动神经末梢。

4. 化学突触：由突触前膜（突触小泡）、突触间隙和突触后膜（受体）组成。

信息传递：化学突触实现神经传导的过程。当神经冲动沿轴膜传导到末端时，细胞外钙离子进入突触前膜，导致突触囊泡移至突触前膜，突触囊泡的膜与突触前膜融合而将递质排出至突触间隙。递质与突触后膜中相应的受体结合，使相应的离子通道开放，突触后膜神经元出现兴奋性突触或者抑制性突触。

Chapter 7　Nervous Tissue

Answer points:

1. Multipolar neurons: Multipolar neurons have one axon but a large number of branching dendrites, such as an anterior horn motor neuron, which has a large cell body, a long axon and several branching dendrites emerging from it. Evenly dispersed Nissl substance can be seen throughout the cell body.

2. Glial cells of CNS: Astrocytes, Oligodendrocytes, Microglia, Ependymal cells; Glial cells of PNS: Schwann cells, Satellite cells.

3. Never endings: Never endings can be classified into sensory nerve endings and motor nerve endings according to their function. The sensory nerve endings are divided into free nerve endings and encapsulated nerve endings. The latter include tactile corpuscle, lamellar corpuscle and muscle spindle. Motor nerve endings are composed of somatic motor nerve endings and visceral motor nerve endings.

4. Chemical synapse: Chemical synapse is composed of presynaptic membrane (synaptic vesicle), synaptic gap and postsynaptic membrand (receptor).

Information transmission: When the conduction of nerve impulses from the axon to the end, the extracellular calcium ions enter the presynaptic membrane, resulting in synaptic vesicles moving to the presynaptic membrane, fusion of the synaptic vesicle membrane with the presynaptic membrane and neurotransmitter is discharged to the synaptic gap. The transmitters combine with the corresponding receptors in the postsynaptic membrane to open the corresponding ion channels and the stimulatory or inhibitory synapses appear in the postsynaptic membrane

第 8 章 神 经 系 统

答题要点：

1. 脊髓是中枢神经的一部分，位于脊椎骨组成的椎管内，呈长圆柱状。脊髓的内部有一个 H 形（蝴蝶型）灰质区，主要由神经细胞构成；在灰质区周围为白质区，主要由有髓神经纤维组成。

2. 小脑皮质分为 3 层，由表及里为：

分子层：少量星形细胞和筐篮细胞；

浦肯野细胞层：浦肯野细胞；

颗粒层：粒细胞、少量高尔基细胞。

3. 大脑皮质一般可分为 6 层，从表面至深层的结构如下。

1）分子层：主要由水平细胞和星形细胞构成。

2）外颗粒层：主要由许多星形细胞和少量小型锥体细胞构成。

3）外锥体细胞层：由许多中、小型锥体细胞和星形细胞组成。

4）内颗粒层：多数是星形细胞。

5）内锥体细胞层：主要由中型和大型锥体细胞组成。

6）多形细胞层：以梭形细胞为主，还有锥体细胞和颗粒细胞。

4. 血 - 脑脊液屏障：由脑内毛细血管内皮细胞、基膜和神经胶质膜构成。

Chapter 8　Nervous System

Answer points:

1. The spinal cord is part of the central nervous system, located in the spinal canal consisting of the vertebrae, and is long cylindrical. Inside the spinal cord, there is an H shaped (butterfly type) gray matter area which is mainly composed of nerve cells. The gray matter area is surrounded by white matter, which is mainly composed of myelinated nerve fibers.

2. The cerebellar cortex is divided into 3 layers, from the outside to the inside:

1) Molecular layer: a small number of stellate cells and basket cells;

2) Purkinje cell layer: Purkinje's cells;

3) Granular layer: granulocytes, a small number of Golgi cells.

3. The cerebral cortex is generally divided into 6 layers, from the outer to the inner structure as follows:

1) Molecular layer: mainly composed of horizontal cells and astrocytes.

2) Outer granular layer: mainly composed of many astrocytes and small pyramidal cells.

3) Outer pyramidal cell layer: many composed of medium and small pyramidal cells and astrocytes.

4) Inner granular layer: mostly composed of astrocytes.

5) The inner pyramidal cell layer: mainly composed of medium and large pyramidal cells.

6) Pleomorphic cell layer: mainly composed of fusiform cells, as well as pyramidal cells and stellate cells.

4. Blood-Brain Barrier (BBB): Composed of cerebral capillary endothelial cells, basement membrane and neuroglia membrane.

第 9 章　循 环 系 统

答题要点：

1. 中动脉：内弹性膜明显，中膜环形平滑肌多，中膜与外膜厚度相当，中膜与外膜交界处有的可见外弹性膜。中静脉无内弹性膜，中膜环形平滑肌少，外膜比中膜厚，无外弹性膜。

2. 大动脉：中膜含有大量弹性膜，故又称之为弹性动脉。中膜比外膜厚，内弹性膜和中膜弹性膜相连，故内膜与中膜分界不明显。没有明显的外弹性膜。

3. 心脏壁的结构分为：心内膜、心肌膜和心外膜；心内膜：内皮、内皮下层、心内膜下层构成。心室的心内膜下层含有心脏传导系统的分支——浦肯野纤维。浦肯野纤维比一般心肌纤维短而宽，胞质中线粒体和糖原丰富，肌丝较少，位于细胞周边，细胞间有较发达的闰盘相连，能快速传导冲动。

Chapter 9　Cardiovascular System

Answer points:

1. In medium-sized artery, internal elastic lamina is prominent. There are more circumferential smooth muscle cells in tunica media. Tunica media and tunica adventitia are similar in thickness. Sometimes an external elastic lamina can be found between tunica media and tunica adventitia. In medium-sized vein, there is no internal elastic lamina. There are less circumferential smooth muscle cells in tunica media. Tunica adventitia is thicker than tunica media. No external elastic lamina can be found.

2. There are numerous elastic laminae in the tunica media of large artery, so large artery is also called elastic artery. In large artery, tunica media is thicker than tunica adventitia. Internal elastic lamina is continuous with elastic laminae in tunica media, so there is no distinct separation between tunica intima and tunica media. No prominent external elastic lamina can be found.

3. The wall of the heart contains endocardium, myocardium and epicardium. The endocardium consists of endothelium, subendothelial layer and subendocardial layer. In ventricle, the subendocardial layer contains Purkinje fibers, the branch of cardiac conduction system. Purkinje fiber is shorter and thicker than typical cardiac muscle cell. It is rich in mitochondria and glycogens in the cytoplasm. Only a few peripherally located myofibrils can be found with in Purkinje cells. Large amount of intercalated disks are present among Purkinje fibers. They assist in the efficient conduction of the heart contraction.

第 10 章　免 疫 系 统

答题要点：

1. 胸腺、副皮质区和动脉周围淋巴鞘。

2. 淋巴小结是球形结构，可见生发中心和小结帽。弥散淋巴组织内可见高内皮微静脉。

3. 淋巴结表面为薄层结缔组织被膜。淋巴结的实质分为皮质和髓质。皮质由浅层皮质、副皮质区和皮质淋巴窦构成。髓质由髓索和髓窦构成。淋巴结的功能为滤过淋巴液和参与机体免疫反应。脾表面为较厚的结缔组织被膜，内含平滑肌。脾的实质分为白髓、红髓和边缘区。白髓由淋巴小结和动脉周围淋巴鞘构成。红髓由脾索和脾血窦构成。脾的功能为造血、贮血、清除衰老红细胞及参与免疫反应。

Chapter 10   Immune System

Answer points:

1. T-cells differentiate and mature in thymus. In peripheral lymphatic organs, T-cells are located mostly in paracortex zone and periarterial lymphatic sheaths.

2. The lymphoid nodule is spherical in shape. Germinal center and dark-staining cap can be found in some lymphoid nodules. High endothelial venule can be found in diffuse lymphoid tissue.

3. The lymph node is covered by thin connective tissue capsule. The parenchyma of lymph node consists of cortex and medulla. The cortex is composed of superficial cortex, paracortex zone and cortical sinus. The medulla is composed of medullary cord and medullary sinus. The lymph node filters lymph and assists the immune system in building an immune response. The spleen is covered by dense connective tissue capsule with smooth muscle cells. The parenchyma of spleen consists of white pulp, red pulp and marginal zone. The white pulp is composed of lymphoid nodule and periarterial lymphatic sheath. The red pulp is composed of splenic cord and splenic sinus. The spleen takes part in hemopoiesis, holds a reserve of blood, removes old red blood cells, and assists the immune system in building an immune response.

第 11 章   皮   肤

答题要点：

1. 毛发由毛干、毛囊、毛球及毛乳头组成。

1）毛干：为长柱形角质蛋白细丝，由内中外三层组成。

a）内层：位于毛发中心，称髓质。

b）中层：称皮质，为毛发构造的主要部分，在电子显微镜下观察，皮质细胞有张力细丝和纤维间基质，细丝由纤维蛋白组成，基质则由富含胱氨酸的非螺丝蛋白组成。

c）外层：又叫毛小皮。位于毛干的最外层，在毛干的基部，起初为一层柱状上皮细胞，逐渐变为长扁平状多层排列，毛小皮细胞在近毛囊上 1/3 处才完全角化。

2）毛囊：也称毛孔。通常每个毛囊内长一根头发，毛囊开口在皮肤的表面，底部深入真皮及皮下脂肪层。每个毛囊都和一个或多个腺泡相连，然后通过腺导管将腺胞离解富含脂质的分泌物运送到皮肤表面排出。

3）毛球：位于毛发根部，是最宽大的部分，是一种增殖能力和分化潜能很强的细胞群。

4）毛乳头：位于毛球基端，为毛发生长提供营养，也称毛基质，主要含两种细胞成分。一种为毛母质细胞，该细胞通过不断分裂分化，增殖向上推移来促使头发生长；另一种是黑色素细胞，其通过不断地分泌色素细胞来决定头发的颜色。

2. 指皮和背皮的结构区别：

不同点	表皮	真皮	角质层	基底层色素颗粒	神经末梢	毛发
指皮	厚	薄	厚	较少	较多	没有
背皮	薄	厚	薄	较多	较少	有

Chapter 11　Skin

Answer points:

1. Hair is composed of hair shaft, hair follicle, hair bulb and dermal papilla.

1) Hair shaft: long columnar keratin filaments, consisting of three layers from inside to outside:

a) Inner layer: it is located in the center of hair, called the medulla.

b) The middle layer: also is called cortex. It is the main part of the hair structure. Under the electron microscope, the cortical cells have tension filaments and inter-fiber matrix. The filaments are made up of fibrin and the matrix is composed of non-spiral proteins rich in cystine.

c) Outer layer: Called caticulapili at the outermost layer of hairy stem, at the base of the hairy stem, the first layer of columnar epithelial cells gradually changes into a long flattened multilayer arrangement. The small hair cells are completely keratinized only at upper 1/3 near the hair follicle.

2) Hair follicle: also called pore. Usually there is one hair in each hair follicle. The hair follicle opens on the surface of the skin, and the bottom goes deep into the dermis and subcutaneous fat layer. Each hair follicle is connected to one or more acini and then transport their lipid rich secretions through the gland ducts.

3) Hair ball: at the root of hair, it is the most extensive part, and is a cell group with strong proliferation and differentiation potential.

4) Hair papilla: at the base of the hair ball, it provides nutrition for hair growth, also known as hair matrix, mainly containing two kinds of cell components. One is the hair generating cells, which is in continuous division and proliferation to promote the growth of hair; the other is melanocytes, which determine the color of hair by continuously secreting pigment.

2. The difference between finger skin and dorsal skin

Difference	Epidermis	Dermis	cuticle layer	Pigment cells in basal layer	Nerve ends	Hair
Finger skin	thick	thin	thick	few	more	no
Dorsal skin	thin	thick	thin	more	few	few

第 12 章　内分泌系统

答题要点：

1. 甲状腺滤泡上皮细胞为立方形，包绕在滤泡周围。细胞核圆形，位于细胞中央。滤泡上皮细胞的高度随着腺体的功能状态而变化，功能活跃时，滤泡上皮细胞增高，呈柱状；反之，滤泡上皮细胞变低呈扁平状。甲状腺滤泡上皮细胞可合成和分泌甲状腺激素。

2. 肾上腺皮质较厚，位于表层，从外往里依次为：球状带、束状带和网状带。

1）球状带细胞：细胞呈低柱状或立方形，排列成球形细胞团，核小而圆，染色深，胞质少，弱嗜碱性，含少量脂滴。分泌盐皮质激素，主要是醛固酮。

2）束状带细胞：由多边形的细胞排列成束；细胞体积大，胞核染色浅，位于中央；胞质内充满脂滴。分泌糖皮质激素，主要是皮质醇。

3）网状带细胞：细胞排列成不规则的条索状，交织成网；细胞较束状带的小，胞核亦小，染色深，胞质弱嗜酸性；含有少量脂滴和较多脂褐素。主要分泌性激素，如脱氢雄酮和雌二醇，也能分泌少量的糖皮质激素。

肾上腺髓质：髓质位于肾上腺的中央部，周围有皮质包绕，上皮细胞排列成索，吻合成网，细胞索间有毛细血管和小静脉。分泌肾上腺素和去甲肾上腺素。

3. 腺垂体远侧部的腺细胞排列成团索状，少数围成小滤泡，细胞间有丰富的毛细血管和少量结缔组织。依据腺细胞着色的差异，可将其分为嗜色细胞和嫌色细胞两大类。嗜色细胞又分为嗜酸性细胞和嗜碱性细胞两种。嗜酸性细胞：生长激素细胞、催乳激素细胞；嗜碱性细胞：促甲状腺激素细胞、促性腺激素细胞、促肾上腺皮质激素细胞。

4. 神经垂体主要由无髓神经纤维和神经胶质细胞组成，含有较丰富的毛细血管。

神经垂体的无髓神经纤维来自下丘脑视上核与室旁核的神经内分泌细胞的轴突。经过漏斗进入神经垂体的神经部，组成下丘脑神经垂体束。神经胶质细胞又称垂体细胞。神经垂体是下丘脑激素的储存和释放部位，因此两者是结构和功能的统一体。

5. 垂体血液供应：主要由垂体上动脉和垂体下动脉供给血液。垂体上动脉从结节部上端伸入神经垂体的漏斗，然后分支，并吻合形成襻状的毛细血管网，称为第一级毛细血管网。这些毛细血管网汇集形成数条垂体门微静脉，下行进入远侧部，再度形成窦状毛细血管，称为第二级毛细血管网。垂体门微静脉及其两端的毛细血管网共同构成垂体门脉

Chapter 12　Endocrine System

Answer points:

1. Thyroid follicular epithelial cells are cubic and wrap around the follicles. The nucleus is round and in the center of the cell. The height of follicular epithelial cells varies with the functional state of glands. The follicular epithelial cells are columnar when they are active. Otherwise, follicular epithelial cells become flat. Thyroid follicle epithelial cells can synthesize and secrete thyroid hormones.

2. The adrenal cortex is thicker and located on the surface of adrenal, which is divided into three layers:

1) Zona glomerulosa: the cells are low columnar or cuboidal, arranged in globular clusters. The nuclei are small and round, deep staining. The cytoplasm is scant, weak basophilia, with a small amount of lipid droplets. The steroids made by these cells are mineralocorticoids, predominantly aldosterone.

2) Zona fasciculata: the polygonal cells are arranged into bundles. The cells are large. The nuclei are in the center, light-stained, and the cytoplasm is filled with lipid droplets. Cells of this zone secrete glucocorticoids, mainly cortisol.

3) Zona reticularis: the cells are arranged in irregular cords, woven into a net. Compared with cells of the zona fasciculata, the nuclei are small, deep stained, with weakly eosinophilic cytoplasm, containing a small amount of lipid droplets and greasy brown pigment. The main secretory hormones are sex hormones, such as dehydroandrosterone, estradiol and a small amount of glucocorticoids.

Adrenal medulla: Medulla lies in the central part of the adrenal gland, surrounded by cortex. The epithelial cells are arranged into cords, forming network. There are capillaries and venules between the cell cords. Epinephrine and norepinephrine are secreted.

3. The main component of the pars distalis are cords of epithelial cells interspersed with rich capillaries and a small amount of connective tissue. Two broad groups of cells in the pars distalis are present based on staining affinity: chromophils and chromophobes. Chromophils are also divided into basophils and acidophils according to their affinity for basic or acidic dyes. Acidophils include somatotropic and mammotropic cells, while the basophilic cells are the thyrotropic cells, gonadotrophic cells, and corticotropic cells.

4. The neurohypophysis is mainly composed of unmyelinated nerve fibers and glial cells, with abundant capillaries. The unmyelinated nerve fibers of the neurohypophysis are the axons of the neuroendocrine neuron which come from the supraoptic nucleus and the paraventricular nucleus. The funnel enters the nerve part of the neurohypophysis and forms the neurohypophysis bundle of the hypothalamus. The glial cells are also known as pituitary cells. The neurohypophysis is the storage and release site of hypothalamic hormones, so they are the unity of structure and function.

5. The blood supply of pituitary gland derives from the superior hypophyseal artery and the inferior hypophyseal artery. The superior hypophyseal artery extends from the upper part of the tubercle to the funnel of the hypophysis, then branches and anastomoses to form the loop-shaped capillary network, which is called the first capillary network. These capillary networks collect and form a number of pituitary portal venules, descending into the far side, forming sinus capillaries again, called the second capillary network. The pituitary portal venule and the capillary networks at both ends constitute the hypophyseal portal system.

第13章 消 化 管

答题要点:

1. 消化管管壁由4层构成: 黏膜层、黏膜下层、肌层、外膜。黏膜层变化最明显。

2. 食管壁分4层结构,上皮为复层扁平上皮,黏膜下层中有食管腺。肌层中可能看见平滑肌和骨骼肌。

3. 小肠表面有绒毛,绒毛根部有小肠腺,小肠上皮中可见柱状吸收细胞和杯状细胞,小肠腺底部可见帕内特细胞。十二指肠黏膜下层有十二指肠腺。

胃表面有胃小凹,上皮为黏液上皮,无杯状细胞,固有层有大量胃底腺,其中壁细胞和主细胞明显,肌层较厚。

结肠表面无绒毛,固有层中含大量大肠腺,杯状细胞多。

Chapter 13   Digestive Tract

Answer points:

1. The wall of the digestive tract contains 4 layers: mucosa, submucosa, muscularis propria and adventitia. The mucosa varies most.

2. The esophageal wall contains 4 layers. The epithelium is stratified squamous epithelium. Esophageal glands are present in submucosa. The muscularis propria contains both skeletal and smooth muscle fibers.

3. The inner surface of small intestine has villi. There are small intestinal glands at the base of villi. In the epithelium, columnar absorptive cells and goblet cells can be found, while Paneth cells can be found at the basal part of small intestinal glands. There are duodenal glands in the submucosa of duodenum.

The inner surface of stomach has gastric pits. The epithelium is mucous epithelium, with no goblet cells. There are many fundic glands in lamina propria. In fundic glands, chief cells and parietal cells are prominent. The muscularis propria is thick.

The inner surface of colon contains no villus. There are many large intestinal glands in lamina propria. Many goblet cells can be found.

第 14 章   消 化 腺

答题要点：

1. 腮腺为纯浆液性腺，闰管长，纹状管较短。分泌物含唾液淀粉酶多，黏液少。颌下腺为混合腺，浆液性腺泡多，黏液性和混合性腺泡少。闰管短，纹状管发达。分泌物含唾液淀粉酶较少，黏液较多。舌下腺为混合腺，以黏液和混合性腺泡为主，浆液性半月形细胞较多，无闰管，纹状管也较短。分泌物以黏液为主。

2. 腮腺是浆液性腺体，实质中含浆液性腺泡和导管。胰腺包括外分泌部和内分泌部。外分泌部含浆液性腺泡和导管，并可见泡心细胞。内分泌部称胰岛，是腺泡之间淡染的细胞团。

3. 肝小叶由中央静脉、肝索、肝血窦、窦周隙、胆小管组成。光镜下 HE 染色标本中窦周隙和胆小管显示不清，两者均可用电镜技术显示，胆小管可经特殊染色后用光镜观察。

Chapter 14   Digestive Gland

Answer points

1. The parotid gland is a serous gland, with long intercalated ducts and short striated ducts. Its secretion contains more salivary amylase and less mucus. The submandibular gland is a mixed gland. It has more serous acini, less mucous and seromucous acini. The intercalated ducts are short. The striated ducts are abundant. Its secretion contains less salivary amylase and more mucus. The sublingual gland is a mixed gland, containing many mucous and seromucous acini. There is no intercalated duct. The striated ducts are short. Its secretion is mainly mucus.

2. The parotid gland is a serous gland. There are many serous acini and ducts in its parenchyma. Pancreas contains both exocrine and endocrine parts. The exocrine pancreas consists of serous acini and ducts, with centroacinar cells. The endocrine pancreas is also called pancreatic islets which are

light-staining cell clusters scattered among the serous acini.

3. The hepatic lobule consists of central vein, hepatic cord, hepatic sinusoid, the space of Disse and bile canaliculus. In HE staining section, the space of Disse and bile canaliculus cannot be identified under light microscope. They can be identified under electron microscope. The bile canaliculus can be identified under light microscope only after special staining.

第 15 章 呼 吸 系 统

答题要点：

1. 肺泡隔是指相邻肺泡之间的间质，其内含有丰富的毛细血管网、大量的弹性纤维及成纤维细胞、肺巨噬细胞和肥大细胞等多种细胞。

功能：隔内丰富的弹性纤维有助于保持肺泡的弹性；肺泡隔内丰富的毛细血管内血液所携带的 CO_2 与肺泡腔内的 O_2 之间进行气体交换所形成的气血屏障。

2. 主要包括：鼻腔前庭部的鼻毛，可阻挡吸入气体中的尘埃颗粒；鼻腔黏膜部的加温过滤功能；从鼻腔直到终末细支气管的黏膜都有纤毛上皮细胞，细胞上的纤毛有利于异物与黏液混合物的排出；黏膜层的杯状细胞和黏液腺分泌的黏液，形成凝胶层以利于黏附异物颗粒。肺泡间隔的尘细胞具有吞噬微生物功能。当各种原因如微生物感染，物理化学因素刺激等导致防御功能降低时，均可导致呼吸系统的损伤。

Chapter 15   Respiratory System

Answer points:

1. The alveolar septum is the interstitium between adjacent alveoli, which contains abundant capillary network, a large number of elastic fibers, fibroblasts, macrophages and mast cells etc.

Function: the abundant elastic fibers in the septa help maintain the elasticity of alveoli. The CO_2 carried by blood in alveolar septum and the O_2 in alveolar cavity go through air-blood barriers in the process of gas exchange.

2. The parts mainly include: the nose hair in nasal vestibule can prevent the dust particles to be inhaled；the warming and filtering function of the nasal mucosa；from the nasal cavity to the terminal bronchioles, the mucosa is lined by ciliated epithelial cells and cilia help dispel foreign particles. Moreover, goblet cells and mucus glands produce mucus secretions, which help adhere the foreign particles. The dust cells in the alveolar septum have the function of phagocytosis. A variety of reasons such as microbial infection, physical and chemical stimulation and so on can lead to the decrease of defense function and damage the respiratory system.

第 16 章 泌 尿 系 统

答题要点：

1. 肾皮质有许多肾小体，肾小体周围有许多近曲小管和远曲小管的断面。肾髓质内有密集排列的肾小管和集合小管。

2. 膀胱壁分黏膜，肌层和外膜三层。黏膜由上皮和固有层构成，上皮为变移上皮。肌层为数层平滑肌。外膜由结缔组织构成。

3. 输尿管管壁由内向外分黏膜，肌层及外膜。各层结构与膀胱类似，但肌层较薄。

Chapter 16   Urinary System

Answer points:

1. The cortex of kidney contains many renal corpuscles. Adjacent to the renal corpuscles are proximal convoluted tubules and distal convoluted tubules. The medulla of kidney consists of renal tubules and collecting tubules.

2. The wall of urinary bladder consists of mucosa, muscularis and adventitia. The mucosa is composed of epithelium and lamina propria. The epithelium is transitional epithelium. The muscularis is composed of several layers of smooth muscle. The adventitia is composed of connective tissue.

3. The wall of ureter consists of mucosa, muscularis and adventitia from inside to outside, which are similar to those of urinary bladder, except that the muscularis is thinner.

第 17 章   男性生殖系统

答题要点：

1. 人的精子是在睾丸中形成的。睾丸里有许多弯弯曲曲的曲细精管。曲细精管中有大量的精原细胞。精原细胞是原始的雄性生殖细胞，每个精原细胞中染色体数目都与体细胞的相同。当雄性动物性成熟时，睾丸里的一部分精原细胞就开始进行减数分裂。经过两次连续的细胞分裂——减数第一次分裂、减数第二次分裂再经过精细胞的变形，就形成了成熟的雄性生殖细胞——精子。

2. 睾丸间质细胞又称 Leydig 细胞，成群分布于生精小管之间的疏松结缔组织内，体积较大，圆形或多边形，核圆，居中，胞质嗜酸性较强。电镜下，具有类固醇激素分泌细胞的超微结构特点，即胞质内含有丰富的滑面内质网、管状嵴的线粒体和较多的脂滴。功能：合成和分泌雄激素，促进精子发生和男性生殖器官的发育，以维持第二性征和性功能。

3. 精子的结构可分为头、颈和尾 3 部分。

1）头部主要由细胞核和顶体组成，呈圆球形、长柱形、螺旋形、梨形和斧形等，这些形状都是由核和顶体的形状决定的。成熟精子的细胞核含有高度致密的染色质，在光学显微镜和电子显微镜下都难以区分其结构。核的前端有顶体，是由双层膜组成的帽状结构覆盖在核的前 2/3 部分，靠近质膜的一层称为顶体外膜，靠近核的一层称为顶体内膜。顶体内有水解酶性质的颗粒，它与精子通过卵外各种卵膜有关。在顶体和核之间的空腔称为顶体下腔，内含肌动蛋白。

2）颈部最短。位于头部以后，呈圆柱状或漏斗状，又称为连接段。它前接核的后端，后接尾部。在前端有基板，由致密物质组成，刚好陷于核后端称为植入窝的凹陷之中。基板之后有一稍厚的头板，两者之间有透明区，其中的细纤维通过基板接连于核后端的核膜。在头板之后为近端中心粒，它虽然稍有倾斜，但与其后的远端中心粒所形成的轴丝几乎垂直。围着这些结构有九条由纵行纤维组成的显示深浅间隔的分节柱，线粒体分布在分节柱的外围。这九条分节柱与其后的 9 条粗纤维的头端紧密相连。

3）尾部分为 3 部分：中段、主段和末段。主要结构是中央的轴丝。

a）中段：从远端中心粒到环之间称为中段，其长度在哺乳类中差异颇大，但结构大体相似。主要结构是轴丝和外围的线粒体鞘。

b）主段：尾部最长的部分，由轴丝和其外的筒状纤维鞘组成。纤维鞘中有两条纤维突起成纵行嵴，由于纵行嵴刚好分别位于背腹二侧，以致使精子尾部截面呈卵圆形。

c）末段：随主段进入末段，纤维鞘逐渐变细而消失。

Chapter 17　Male Reproductive System

Answer points:

1. Human sperm is formed in the testicles. There are many curved seminiferous tubules in the testicles, called seminiferous tubules. There are a large number of spermatogonia cells in the seminiferous tubules. Spermatogonias are primitive male germ cells. The number of chromosomes in each spermatogonia is the same as that of somatic cells. When male animals mature, some spermatogonia begin to undergo meiosis. After two successive cell divisions-the first meiosis division, the second meiosis division, and the deformations of the spermatocyte, forming the mature male germ cells—sperms are formed.

2. The interstitial cells of the testis, also known as Leydig cells, are distributed in loose connective tissue among the seminiferous tubules, with large size, round or polygonal, centrally located round nuclei and strong eosinophilic cytoplasm. Under electron microscope, it has the ultrastructural characteristics of the steroid hormone producing cells, that is, the cytoplasm contains abundant smooth surface endoplasmic reticulum, mitochondria of tubular crista and more lipid droplets. Function: synthesis and secretion of androgen, promoting spermatogenesis and male reproductive organ development, so as to maintain secondary sexual characteristics and sexual functions.

3. the structure of spermatozoa can be divided into 3 parts: head, neck and tail.

1) The head is mainly composed of the nucleus and acrosome, which can be round, columnar, spiral, pear and axe etc. All of which are determined by the shape of the nucleus and the acrosome. The nuclei of mature spermatozoa contain highly dense chromatin, which is difficult to distinguish under optical microscope or electron microscope. The front of the nucleus is an acrosome, a double layer of cap that covers the first 2/3 parts of the nucleus. One layer near the plasma membrane is called the apical outer membrane, and the layer near the nucleus is called the endorum. There are particles with hydrolytic enzymes in the apical body, which are involved in sperm going through various membranes outside the egg. The cavity between the acrosome and the nucleus is sub-acrosomal cavity, containing actin.

2) Neck is the shortest portion. After the head, it is cylindrical or funnel-shaped, also known as the connecting segment. It connects the rear end of the core and the tail. There are substrates at the front end, made up of dense materials and just trapped in the rear end of the cavity, like a dent in the socket. There is a thicker head plate behind the substrate, and there is a transparent area between them. The fine fibers are connected to the nuclear membrane at the back end of the nucleus through the substrate. After the head plate is the proximal centrosome, although it is slightly tilted, it is almost perpendicular to the axis filament formed by the distal centrosome. Surrounding these structures, there are nine vertical columns separated by segmental fibers, and the mitochondria are distributed around the outside of those segmental columns. These nine columns are closely linked to

the top end of the 9 coarse fibers.

3) The tail is divided into 3 parts: the middle, the main and the last. The main structure is the shaft of the central axis.

a) The middle part: from the distal centrosome to the ring, it is called the middle part, and its length is quite different in mammals, but its structure is similar. The main structure is the axoneme and the mitochondrial sheath.

b) Main segment: the longest part of the tail consists of a axoneme and its outer cylindrical fibrous sheath. The fibrous sheath has two fibers protruding into longitudinal crests. The two longitudinal crests lie on each dorsal and ventral side, so that the section of the sperm tail is oval.

c) The end piece: with the main segment entering the end, the fibrous sheath gradually becomes thin and disappears.

第 18 章　女性生殖系统

答题要点：

1. 卵泡由卵母细胞和卵泡细胞组成。卵泡发育是个连续的生长过程，其结构发生一系列变化，一般可分为原始卵泡、初级卵泡、次级卵泡和成熟卵泡四个阶段。

1）原始卵泡：原始卵泡位于皮质浅部，体积小，数量多。卵泡中央有一个初级卵母细胞，周围为单层扁平的卵泡细胞（又称颗粒细胞）。初级卵母细胞圆形，较大，直径约 40μm，核大而圆，染色质疏，着色浅，核仁大而明显，胞质嗜酸性。

2）初级卵泡：此时期的初级卵母细胞体积增大，细胞核变大；卵泡细胞由单层扁平变为立方形或柱状，细胞层数增殖成多层。在卵母细胞和卵泡细胞之间出现透明带。

3）次级卵泡：卵泡体积更大，卵泡细胞增至 6～12 层，细胞间出现一些不规则的腔隙，并逐渐合并成一个较大的卵泡腔，腔内充满卵泡液。随着卵泡液的增多及卵泡腔扩大，卵母细胞居于卵泡的一侧，并与其周围的颗粒细胞一起突向卵泡腔，形成卵丘。此时初级卵母细胞直径可达 125～150μm。紧贴透明带的一层柱状卵泡细胞呈放射状排列，称放射冠。分布在卵泡腔周边的卵泡细胞较小，构成卵泡壁，称为颗粒层。在卵泡生长过程中，卵泡膜分化为内、外两层。内膜层含有较多的多边形或梭形的膜细胞及丰富的毛细血管。外膜层主要由结缔组织构成，胶原纤维较多，并含有平滑肌纤维。

4）成熟卵泡：卵泡体积很大，直径可达 20mm，并向卵巢表面突出。成熟卵泡的卵泡腔很大，颗粒层很薄，颗粒细胞也不再增殖。此时的初级卵母细胞又恢复成熟分裂，在排卵前 36～48 小时完成第一次成熟分裂。产生 1 个次级卵母细胞和 1 个很小的第一极体。第一极体位于次级卵母细胞和透明带之间的卵周间隙内。次级卵母细胞随即进入第二次成熟分裂，停止于分裂中期。

2. 排卵后卵泡壁向腔内塌陷，颗粒层细胞和膜细胞发育为黄体，结缔组织和毛细血管长入，最外层形成结缔组织膜，新鲜时显黄色，称为黄体。由颗粒细胞分化来的黄体细胞为颗粒黄体细胞，数量多，细胞大，着色浅，位于黄体中央，分泌孕激素。膜细胞分化来的黄体细胞称为膜黄体细胞，细胞小，染色深，大部位于黄体外周，分泌雌激素。若卵子受精，在人绒毛膜促性腺激素的作用下，黄体继续增长，至妊娠 6 个月甚至更长时间后慢慢萎缩，成为妊娠黄体。若卵子未受精，黄体维持 2 周后便退化，称为月经黄体。被结缔组织结瘢所代替，即白体。

Chapter 18   Female Reproductive System

Answer points:

1. The follicle is composed of oocyte and follicular cell. Follicular development is a continuous growth process. Its structure has undergone a series of changes. It can be generally divided into four stages: primordial follicle, primary follicle, secondary follicle and mature follicle.

1) The primordial follicle: Primordial follicle is located in the superficial cortex, with small volume and a large number of follicles. There is a primary oocyte at the center of the follicle, surrounded by a single layer of flat follicle cells (also known as granulosa cells). Primary oocyte is round and large, with a diameter of about 40 μm, large and round nucleus, thin chromatin, lightly stained, large and prominent nucleoli and eosinophilic cytoplasm.

2) The primary follicle: The primary oocyte and its nuclei increase in size at this stage. The follicle cells change from single flattened layer to multi-layers of cuboidal or columnar cells. The zona pellucida occurs between oocyte and follicle cells.

3) The secondary follicle: The volume of follicle continues to grow and the follicle cells increase to 6-12 layers. There are irregular lacunae among cells and are gradually merged into a large follicle cavity, which filled with follicular fluid. During the reorganization of the granulosa layer to form the antrum, some cells form a small hillock, called the cumulus oophorus, surrounding the oocyte and protruding into the antrum. At this time the primary oocyte diameter can reach 125-150μm. A layer of columnar follicle cells that cling to the zona pellucida is radially arranged, called the corona radiata. The follicle cells around the follicle cavity are smaller and form the follicle wall, called stratum granulosum. In the process of follicle growth, the follicular membrane is divided into two layers, interna and externa. The theca interna contains more polygonal and spindle-shaped theca cells and rich in capillaries. The theca externa is mainly composed of connective tissue, with more collagen fibers and smooth muscle fibers.

4) The mature follicles: The volume of the follicle is large at this stage. The diameter of the follicle is up to 20mm, and it is protruding to the surface of the ovary. The follicle cavity of the mature follicle is very large. The granulosa layer becomes very thin, and the granulosa cells no longer proliferate. The primary oocyte at this time resumes meiotic division and completes the first meiosis at 36-48 hours before ovulation. A secondary oocyte and a very small first polar body are produced. The first polar body is located in the perivitelline space between the secondary oocyte and the zona pellucida. The secondary oocyte immediately enters the second meiotic division and stops in the middle of the division.

2. The follicle wall collapses into the cavity after ovulation, and the granulosa cells and theca cells develop into corpus luteum. Connective tissue and capillaries grow into the outer layer, forming connective tissue membrane. It is yellow when fresh, called corpus luteum. The corpus luteum cells differentiated from granulosa cells are granulosa lutein cells. They are abundant large cells, lightly stained, located in the central part of corpus luteum and secrete progesterone. The of corpus luteum cells differentiated from the theca cells are called theca lutein cells. They are small cells with deep staining, mostly located at the periphery of corpus luteum and secrete estrogen. If the egg

is fertilized, under the action of human chorionic gonadotropin, the corpus luteum will continue to grow, until about 6 months of pregnancy or even longer, and become the corpus luteum of pregnancy before its atrophy. If the egg is not fertilized, the corpus luteum is degenerated after about two weeks, which is called the corpus luteum of menstruation, which will in turn be replaced by connective tissue scarring, namely corpus albicans.

第 19 章　眼　和　耳

答题要点：

角膜的组织结构分 5 层：角膜上皮、前界膜、角膜基质、后界膜和角膜内皮。

其主要透明因素：上皮不角化，无色素，固有层无血管，胶原纤维粗细均一，排列规律，水分恒定等。

Chapter 19　Eye and Ear

Answer points:

Cornea consists of five layers: corneal epithelium, anterior limiting lamia, corneal stroma, posterior limiting lamina, and corneal endothelium.

The transparent characteristics of the cornea: corneal epithelium is nonkeratinized stratified squamous epithelium without chromocyte; corneal stroma contains collagen fibers, which are uniform in diameter and have a unique pattern—regularly arranged, parallel in each layer and at right angle in successive layers; the stroma contains stable water content, and has no blood vessels.

（任芳丽　郭晓霞）

参 考 文 献
References

［1］李和，李继承. 组织学与胚胎学［M］. 3 版. 北京：人民卫生出版社，2015.

［2］唐军民，李英，卫兰. 组织学与胚胎学彩色图谱（实习用书）［M］. 2 版，北京：北京大学医学出版社，2013.

［3］唐军民，张雷. 组织学与胚胎学［M］. 3 版. 北京：北京大学医学出版社，2013.

［4］ANTHONY L, MESCHER. Junqueira's basic histology text & atlas [M]. McGraw-Hill Education, 2013.

英 - 中文组织学名词索引
English–Chinese Histological Nouns Index